Staffing:
A Journal of
Nursing Administration Reader

Staffing:
A Journal of
Nursing Administration Reader

Selected by
Mary Ellen Warstler, R.N., M.A.
Director Department of Nursing Services
American Nurses' Association
Kansas City, Missouri
Contemporary Publishing, Inc. Wakefield Massachusetts

Copyright © 1974 by Contemporary Publishing, Inc. Wakefield, Massachusetts

First edition

Library of Congress Catalog Card Number: 74-76942
International Standard Book Number: 0-913654-01-9

Type set by WILLIAMS GRAPHIC SERVICE, INC.

Manufactured in the United States of America
by WILLIAM BYRD PRESS Richmond, Virginia

STAFFING:
Table of Contents

1 Primary Nursing: An Organization
That Promotes Promotional Practice
Karen L. Ciske

4 Staffing for Quality Care
Myrtle K. Aydelotte

8 Some Management Techniques
For Nursing Service Administrators
Mary Ellen Warstler

18 Cyclic Work Schedules and
a Nonnurse Coordinator of Staffing
Mary Ellen Warstler

24 The Reconstructed Work Week:
One Answer to the Scheduling Dilemma
Lorraine P. Fraser

29 Clinical Staffing With a 10-Hour Day,
4-Day Work Week
Jeannine Bauer

31 Community Nursing Administration:
Quantify Nursing Utilization
Charmaine L. Kissinger

37 Satisfaction of Job Factors
for Registered Nurses
Douglas A. Benton and Harold C. White

45 Job Satisfaction and Float Assignments
Barbara Thomas

52 Maintaining the Job Performance
of the Aging Employee
*Lawrence L. Steinmetz
and R. Dennis Middlemist*

INTRODUCTION

Nursing administrators have an increasing need for references that will help them to evaluate their staffing plans and will provide ideas for updating their present staffing programs.

The American Nurses' Association Nursing Services Department, in the belief that a collection of Staffing articles from *The Journal of Nursing Administration* would be one means for meeting the urgent need for references, initiated the process that led to publication of this book by Contemporary Publishing.

As the federal government presses for more rigid monetary control over health agencies, the nursing budget receives closer scrutiny in efforts to reduce general patient care costs. Therefore the struggle between cost savings and the provision of quality patient care grows more intense. Nursing administrators are consequently forced to look more closely for overlapping schedules and poor distribution of personnel in relation to the day-to-day needs for patient care. Another concern is the impact on costs of the productivity level of nursing personnel. Can nursing administrators continue to allow non-nursing functions to be carried by nursing care personnel?

Not all the answers are found with this book, but many useful ideas and tools are described and some of the articles have reference lists that will take you further into the available literature.

Mary Ellen Warstler
Kansas City, Missouri
February 1974

Primary Nursing:

An Organization That Promotes Professional Practice

by Karen L. Ciske

Karen L. Ciske, R.N., M.S.N. was Consultant in Rehabilitation Nursing, University of Minnesota Hospitals, Minneapolis, when this article was written. She is now an independent consultant/instructor/facilitator to hospital nursing departments desiring assistance in implementing primary nursing or improving its delivery. The article is reprinted from JONA, January-February 1974.

Hospital nursing has been a difficult place to implement professional practice. In an attempt to find ways to improve the delivery of nursing care and the level of staff satisfaction, a group of nurses at the University of Minnesota Hospitals adapted the one-to-one assignment model to a small patient unit. Decision making was decentralized to the nurse who knew the patient best, the primary nurse. Because of her role in staff development, the head nurse was seen to be pivotal to the success of primary nursing.

The hospital as the agency that employs the majority of practicing nurses in the United States is often the most difficult place in which to practice nursing. Some of the frustrations experienced by staff nurses are reflected in surveys of graduate nurses working in hospitals. Kramer found a 20 percent potential or actual dropout rate from nursing for a group of nurses followed during a two-year period after graduation [1]. She reports that there is a continuing drop in the scores pertaining to professional role conception (beliefs and values about the nursing role), which would imply that nurses become less professional with continued employment [2]. Harrington and Theis and Sister Reinkemeyer also have studied the roles of baccalaureate nurses and point out dissatisfactions pertaining to employment in traditional hospital settings [3, 4].

Why does this situation exist? I believe it is because many hospitals tend to be bureaucratic organizations that place value on efficiency, predictability, rules, and authority. Malone has done a masterful job of describing the problem of a professional within a bureaucracy [5]. She suggests changes in the organization of hospital services so that graduate nurses who are committed to professional practice might implement what they have been taught in their educational programs as quality care for their patients. To a great extent this might help to prevent role deprivation resulting in disillusionment, bitterness, adaptation to other values, and unsatisfactory patient care.

With this concern in mind—to somehow make it possible to practice nursing at a higher professional level in our hospital setting—I became involved in 1968 in an experimental project designed to improve the delivery of services to patients on a small medical unit. I was nurse clinician on this unit and several others at the University of Minnesota Hospitals. I worked with other clinicians, administrative supervisors in nursing, inservice staff, head nurses, and faculty from the school of nursing as a member of the steering committee to determine the needs for change and implement them. The following is an overview of the process through which our group and the nursing staff of the 23-bed medical unit accomplished rather dramatic changes in the organization and delivery of nursing care.

One aspect of our project was the development of a ward manager position; another was the examination of existing systems in delivery of care by nursing and other hospital departments. Although we recognized that we might be freeing nurses to nurse by establishing a ward manager role, we were aware that this in itself might not improve patient care. The Iowa study, in 1960, had confirmed that increasing the time devoted to direct patient care had not automatically produced *better* patient care [6]. Thus, we began to examine our organization of nursing services at the unit level.

We were utilizing team nursing on most units, but our particular brand of team nursing seemed to perpetuate deficiencies in the acceptance of responsibility for care planning and follow-through on many of these units. Shared responsibility and accountability often became *no responsibility and accountability*. The team leader's goals of assessing each patient on her team and supervising the planning, implementing, and evaluating of care plans for ten to twenty patients were unmet.

In studying our situation we began to see how unrealistic were our expectations of team leaders. In our busy, acute care hospital we were asking a registered nurse, often newly graduated from any one of three kinds of educational programs and working rotating shifts to: (1) know and act upon the critical information on her patients in order to plan their care, using the team conference whenever appropriate; (2) lead other team members, which involved assigning, supervising and teaching licensed practical nurses, orderlies, and aides; and (3) observe and constantly evaluate the care patients received. From the patient's point of view, care was extremely fragmented with as many as three or four of the nursing staff caring for him during one shift. As a clinician, I found it difficult to help the staff achieve comprehensive care for patients or to find satisfaction in their jobs.

In looking for alternatives to the team-nursing structure, we investigated what other nursing services were doing. For several years Loeb Center for Nursing and Rehabilitation in New York City had been working with organizational patterns other than traditional team or functional nursing. Their patients are assigned to professional nurses who are responsible for and provide the total nursing care throughout the patient's stay. A nurse is assigned a specific "district" of patients and plans with them for the achievement of their health care goals. She cares for them each day she is on duty; thus, continuity is improved with few aspects of the patient's care delegated to nonprofessional workers.

Other examples of this one-to-one assignment can be found in private duty, public health, and psychiatric nursing practices. The principle of a one-to-one assignment in our hospital had previously been adapted successfully to the rehabilitation units and we wondered if this method could succeed on acute care units as well.

The nursing committee described what we wanted to accomplish for patients in a "job description for comprehensive care." The focus was on continuity of nurse-patient relationship wherein the nurse would: (1) encourage the patient to participate in his own care and to express himself; (2) be knowledgeable about the patient's medical condition, personal and family data, and implications for nursing care; (3) teach the patient and work with the family; (4) plan for other staff involvement through the kardex and other communications; and (5) refer the patient to other professionals when appropriate.

Since it seemed somewhat risky to remove the security of the team system before the staff had an opportunity to "try on" these responsibilities and/or learn how to act more independently than they had previously, we asked them to choose and provide care until discharge for a few "comprehensive care patients" in their teams. It was expected that the nurses would try to fulfill the comprehensive care job description, as well as continue their team nursing responsibilities. We introduced a new kardex form with more space for nursing evaluation, weekly classes on the elements of comprehensive care, and the concept of total care. Total care meant that the patient related with one nurse during any given shift for the care required —medications, vital signs, hygiene, treatments, teaching, etc.

After several months of what we perceived as a greater degree of comprehensive care within the team system than formerly, a rising level of staff frustration and anxiety became apparent. Nurses were not selecting patients for comprehensive care, and they were reluctant to write on the kardex or to talk about their plans for their patients. After examining what was happening, we found that we had inadvertently created an even more tense and frustrating situation than before. Team leaders were fulfilling their expected roles as they had before the project, but *in addition* they were trying to follow a few patients for comprehensive care. Because they were committed to its principles and felt unsuccessful in its accomplishment, they seemed to be blaming themselves as being inadequate nurses. The problem was the *system* we had introduced! As the planning and steering committee we had asked nurses to assume greater responsibility for individual patients than they had formerly assumed in team nursing, but we were not relieving them of any of their team-leading tasks.

After discussing this problem at a staff meeting, we made what was to us a momentous decision. We dissolved the team structure and assigned each nurse to a group of patients. We also identified realistic, minimum expectations for kardex information. The "check-up" system within the team was eliminated, and each nurse became responsible and accountable for accomplishing all that was necessary for her assigned patients during her shift. It was understood that the consequences of these changes would be evaluated and that the team or another system could be resumed if necessary.

At this time the label *primary nursing* was adopted. The basic concepts in this system of practice are:

1. Assignment of each patient to a specific (primary) nurse, who usually provides his care each day she is on duty until the patient's discharge or transfer.
2. Patient assessment by the primary nurse, who plans the care to be given when she is not on duty, when secondary or associate nurses care for her patients. Thus, 24-hour responsibility for care is actualized through the primary nurse's written directives on kardex and other communication tools.
3. Patient involvement in the care provided and identification of his goals relating to how the medical condition affects his life style.
4. Care giver to care giver communication—both in the nursing staff's daily reporting methods and between disciplines.
5. Discharge planning—including patient teaching, family involvement, and appropriate referrals.

Primary nursing is often confused with primary care, the latter being the mechanism by which a client enters the health care system. Usually this contact is in the community, and the health professional could be a nurse. However, primary nursing as defined in our project is a system of hospital nursing services at the unit level with the components listed above.

In our experience with primary nursing we have found that the head nurse is the person most qualified to assign nurses to patients according to the care needs of patients and the abilities and/or case load of the staff nurse because, ultimately, she is responsible for the quality of care delivered to the patients on her unit. She is also responsible for evaluating staff and providing opportunities for their development. When the head nurse is aware that the patient's needs are beyond the ability of the primary nurse, she either chooses to work closely with her or assigns a second nurse to assist with specific aspects of the care to be given.

The upgrading of the unit secretary's job, the improvement of support systems (pharmacy, central supply, etc.), and the creation of the departmental assistant, whose functions are similar to those described for ward managers, were important factors contributing to changes in the head nurse and staff roles. Because the head nurse is now less obligated to supervise and perform desk activities, she is able to work more closely with her staff. Consequently, the staff benefit from her knowledge of patient care and gradually become more independent. After eighteen months of primary nursing, many of the head nurse's functions were observed to be consistent with the role of nurse clinician, when examined by Kramer and Manthey [7].

We had anticipated that the RN was the only level of nursing personnel prepared for the responsibilities of primary nursing. Therefore, the head nurse assigned each RN, including herself, to a group of patients. Most staff had three or four patients. However, several LPNs on the staff demonstrated excellent patient care ability and wanted a chance to be a primary nurse. We were reluctant but decided to assign them a patient along with an RN or the head nurse on a trial basis. We worked closely with these LPNs, as well as with many of the less experienced RNs, and were able to help them identify needs for additional skills and/or knowledge. After a few months we found some of the LPNs to be excellent primary nurses for certain patients, well able to establish care plans and make decisions with their patients. Nursing aides were not involved in direct care on some shifts and acted mainly as messengers. When they gave patient care, however, they worked closely with a primary nurse and received better instructions than previously.

Since staff members knew who was assigned to each patient, the quality of nursing care was more visible. An empty kardex versus clearly written instructions for care were evidences of the evaluative efforts and communication ability of the primary nurse. During the time in which the medical unit described has been using the primary nursing system, there have been a number of promotions to head nurse or inservice staff positions. These promotions may have been related to our being better able to *evaluate* the abilities of these nurses; the outcomes of their work with their primary patients were visible. This visibility of nursing judgments was frightening to many of the staff who felt some insecurity about being the main care planner and problem solver for a group of patients. They needed support, instruction, and encouragement.

Group meetings and classes were held on a regular basis. As needs for knowledge were identified, these classes were changed in content from assessment and care planning to a review of the medical diagnoses commonly seen on that unit. What came as a surprise to us was how much anxiety staff felt concerning the expectations of direct communication with the physician and more extensive patient teaching activities. They needed and wanted disease review. Classes on medical conditions and nursing implications were well received and used by the nurses.

There have been some exciting outcomes of our experiment. These are:

1. Staff enthusiasm toward patient care and a feeling of accomplishment with *their* patients.
2. Awareness of the strengths within the group for teaching and supporting each other—staff meetings were held regularly during the first year and periodically as needed.
3. Decrease in the turnover rate of RNs and LPNs.
4. Decrease in patient stereotyping by nurses as "difficult," "demanding," etc. with corresponding decrease in frustration and in staff/patient struggle for control.
5. Patients' and families' gratitude for having one nurse in charge of their care and coordinating other staff efforts.
6. Positive reports from nurses who "float" to primary nursing units.
7. Development of better systems of communicating with agencies following our patients after discharge, e.g., public health nursing, extended care, nursing homes.
8. Ten other units at our hospital have adopted the primary nursing structure.
9. Much interest in primary nursing has been shown by hospitals and schools of nursing in the community.

Many questions are still to be answered. Does the primary nursing system really facilitate the accomplishment of professional nursing as we think it has, or have improvements been related to the attention and support given to the group rather than from the changed organization itself? How can we help the head nurse to assume a different and very demanding role? How can we best develop the staff nurse's abilities and motivation toward functioning in a more independent role than before?

Primary nursing is not a panacea. It will not cure incompetent nursing practices or change staff attitudes about how much of themselves they are willing to give in relationships with patients or with other staff members. It demands knowledge of how to work within change in order to effectively utilize the group as the steps of change occur. And it requires clinical nursing leaders who are available as resources to the staff and head nurse when they face the problems and risks that come from entrusting the primary nurse with responsibility and accountability for patient care decisions.

There are indications from many disciplines that what one makes explicit to people as expectations of behavior affects what they can and will accomplish. This is true of hospital nursing. Our philosophy in primary nursing relates directly to individualizing patient care through a nurse-patient relationship wherein acceptance of responsibility and accountability is *expected*. We feel that professional practice has been promoted through our experience in primary nursing.

REFERENCES

1. Kramer, M. The new graduate speaks again. *Am. J. Nurs.* 69 (9): 1907, 1969.
2. Ibid., p. 1904.
3. Harrington, H., and Theis, E. C. Institutional factors perceived by baccalaureate graduates as influencing their performance as staff nurses. *Nurs. Res.* 13 (3): 228, 1968.
4. Reinkemeyer, Sister A. It won't be hospital nursing! *Am. J. Nurs.* 68 (9): 1936, 1968.
5. Malone, M. F. The dilemma of a professional in a bureaucracy. *Nurs. Forum* 3 (4): 36, 1964.
6. Aydelotte, M. K., and Tener, M. *An Investigation of the Relation between Nursing Activity and Patient Welfare.* State University of Iowa Press, Iowa City, 1960.
7. Manthey, M., and Kramer, M. A dialogue on primary nursing. *Nurs. Forum* 9 (4): 365–366, 1970.

BIBLIOGRAPHY

Manthey, M. Primary nursing is alive and well in the hospital. *Am. J. Nur.* 73 (1): 83, 1973.
Manthey, M., Ciske, K., Robertson, P., and Harris, I. Primary nursing: A return to the Concept of "my nurse" and "my patient." *Nurs. Forum* 9 (1): 65, 1970.

staffing for quality care

by Myrtle K. Aydelotte

Myrtle K. Aydelotte, R.N., Ph.D., is Director of Nursing, University of Iowa Hospitals and Clinics, and Professor at the College of Nursing, Iowa City. The article is reprinted from JONA, March-April 1973.

The major purpose of a department of nursing within a health care delivery system is to provide nursing care to patients. To many nurses and nursing educators this statement may appear unnecessary. However, there apparently is so much confusion about what constitutes adequate nursing care and how it is provided that the Joint Commission on Accreditation of Hospitals (JCAH) in the second part of Standard I explicitly calls attention to the need for sufficient and adequate nursing staff to provide quality care to patients. The second portion of the statement reads: "The nursing service shall be under the direction of a legally and professionally qualified registered nurse and there shall be a sufficient number of registered nurses who are currently licensed in the state on duty at all times to give patients nursing care that requires their judgment and specialized care and to plan, supervise, and evaluate the nurse care of patients" [1].

Information used in interpreting the standard and the data sought as evidence of its presence deal with such topics as staffing allocations, numbers, specific settings, references to characteristics of patients, establishment of goals, and the like. Knowledge about these various factors is important; but in the implementation of action to achieve the standard, the director draws upon background dealing with more concepts than the few alluded to in the manual.

The director of nursing service is charged with the development and execution of a program of staffing. She therefore must have knowledge about the elements of a staffing program and the tools necessary for its planning, implementation, and evaluation. Staffing is a major program of the department, a consideration which most directors and their associates give more attention to than they believe it deserves [2]. The large amount of time spent in staffing is due in part to manpower problems, such as shortages and personnel preferences, but is also greatly due to the lack of conceptualization of the totality of the program, failure to recognize significant variables, and lack of intellectual skills required in the construction of the total program.

A staffing program is made up of four elements:
1. Identification of the quality of the product to be rendered to the client

2. Prediction of the number and kind of personnel needed to produce the volume and quality of nursing care required
3. The selection and arrangement of the nursing staff in specific configurations and the development of assignment patterns for the staff required 24 hours per day, 7 days per week
4. The evaluation of the effectiveness of the staff's product (nursing care) upon the patient population to whom it is rendered

The identification of these elements enables nursing to perceive staffing as something more than "plugging the holes" or "finding the hands and feet" to fill a gap in a staffing pattern. It assists us in seeing that the relationship between patient requirements and staff knowledge and skills is reciprocal. The impact of nursing practice upon patients should result in an effect which can be observed and measured in changes in and around the patient. Consequently, staffing a unit is not a matter of random or careless assignment of nursing personnel. It is the result of deliberate and careful selection of specific individuals and a prediction of their effect upon patients. This prediction is based upon a careful analysis of the requirements of the population to be served and the variables which we believe to be influencing nursing practice.

WHAT IS THE QUALITY OF THE PRODUCT TO BE DELIVERED?

The first decision to be made by the leadership group in a department of nursing service concerns the quality of care to be provided the patients. Consideration of the goal of services is paramount since it sets the parameters to be used in planning staffing. Many variables enter into making the decision about goals and quality. Not only is there the question of compliance with laws and regulations set forth by governmental agencies, but there is also the need to take into account client expectations and the beliefs of the nursing staff as to what is acceptable practice for them to produce. The presence or absence of medical care programs and educational programs, the financial constraints placed upon the community which the hospital serves, the policies and requirements of third party payers, and the extent to which the patient is able to pay for services himself also enter into the often unspoken negotiations between the nursing department's spokesman, the director of nursing, and the hospital administrator as well as between leaders of other departments in the hospital arena.

The question of whether the nursing practice will be directed toward meeting the patient's requirements in full or whether priorities must be established depends upon many factors. The extent to which this question is explored before a decision is made often rests upon the ability to describe the patient care requirements, through precise use of language and "hard data," indicating quantification of evidence. The director's ability to conceptualize the total program of the hospital and its financial base will also determine how well she can present reasonable demands and how effectively she can play her part in assisting the professional and administrative group in arriving at the goals to be set for the hospital. She must be realistic in her evaluation of whether the patients truly require some of the services we have traditionally been taught that patients need. This is not to imply that the director is impersonal and cold. It indicates that she must view the program of nursing service in relation to its value to and its effect upon the patient and the primary purpose for which the patient is being seen by the health professionals.

Therefore, the first task in setting up a staffing program is the development of objectives of nursing care to be achieved by the department of nursing and by the staff on each nursing unit. These objectives should be feasible, attainable, and measurable [3]. Too often the objectives are global and reflect myths and folklore about nursing practice which can neither be described in operational terms nor attained by the staff.

WHAT ARE STAFF METHODOLOGIES?

The nursing workload is dependent upon patient care requirements and is directed toward accomplishment of the objectives established for that care. Staffing requirements for that workload is determined by applying a nurse staffing methodology. Nurse staffing methodology is a systematic process applied to determine the numbers and kinds of nursing personnel required to provide nursing care of a predetermined quality to a specific group of patients. The methodology utilizes selected tools to identify or measure the variables that influence the amount of care required. The process is procedurally arranged and formally documented.

The specific methodology selected may be representative of four general types:
1. Simple descriptive
2. Industrial engineering
3. Management engineering
4. Operations research

The descriptive methodology makes use of a number of data-gathering devices about a large number of variables among which the interaction is not clear. Use is made of simple ratios, formulas, fluctuations of census, proportions of personnel, and judgment based upon common sense and experience. A variety of models are available for use, but there is no consistent strategy.

The industrial methodology is directed at the study of nursing work on a specific unit and focuses more upon reorganization, reassignment, and redistribution of work than on new prediction of total work. It uses techniques of work measurement, task or function analysis, and procedure flow and analysis.

The management engineering methodology utilizes these same tools and techniques, but also draws upon systems analysis and operations research. Its component strategies are seven: (1) a statement of performance objectives; (2) an analysis of components and functions; (3) distribution of functions; (4) scheduling; (5) training of individuals for use and testing of the system; (6) installation of the system; and (7) quality control.

In the operations research methodology, mathematical models are built to test real life problems, using data from the real world. The structures for solutions are explored and procedures are established for obtaining them. Following the tests for solutions, the optimal one is then made available for use.

The decision of which methodology to use rests again upon a number of factors which must be considered by the director and the staff. Among the more important variables operating to influence this decision are these:

1. The definition of nursing practice held by the department
2. The availability of data depicting variables held important
3. The sophistication of the staff and their ability to deal with the methodology
4. The amount of error in prediction of workload which can be allowed
5. The general volume of the number of staff to be dealt with
6. The financial stringency of the operation with which the director of nursing must deal

It is imperative that the limitations of the methodology selected be recognized and specified as the results are interpreted to the staff and the administrator. The extent of our knowledge about staffing methodologies is limited. The research about variables thought to be important to nurse staffing varies greatly in quality. Some studies are excellent; others exceedingly poor. Much of it is not definitive. For example, one cannot say that patients housed in a radially designed unit require less nursing staff than a comparable and equal number of patients cared for in a nursing unit of a double corridor design. Neither can we say that the presence of a unit manager system in a hospital requires less nursing staff, although we think it may. Unfortunately, the research on these important variables has not clearly delineated the knowledge we require to predict their effects upon staffing requirements. We can assume therefore that study of the variables thought to be impinging upon staffing will result in a better judgment about staffing than no consideration of variables. Included among these variables are: (1) patient census, its average and its variation; (2) hospital policies regarding admission and discharge and the handling of emergencies; (3) nursing workload, measured either by application of a patient classification system, or task count and standard time, or both; (4) personnel statistics, personnel policies, and position descriptions; (5) presence or absence of supporting services; (6) attributes of quality of nursing care; (7) definition of nursing practice; and (8) architectural factors, such as design and the presence or absence of supporting services.

Patient classification schemes, which are used fairly extensively in staffing methodologies, possess characteristics of which the director and her staff should be aware. First, the majority of schemes are developed along the physiological dimensions of care primarily; few scales have items related to a given patient's sociopsychological behavior or requirements. Second, little is reported in the literature or in guides about the precision with which patients can be classified. Third, the question of the validity of the terms used in classification schemes has not been resolved to anyone's satisfaction.

The application of any methodology must be viewed in relation to all aspects of the staffing program. The purpose of the methodology is to provide a process by which predictions of staff can be made. The success or failure of a staff in its production lies not alone in numbers, mix, and supporting services. The productivity of a staff resides in the knowledge, skill, and motivation possessed by the individuals on that staff.

The identification of categories of staff to be employed suggests the minimal training required for appointments. Productivity of staff is based upon the interaction of the nursing staff and the means by which it puts its talents to use. It is upon the leadership group that the motivation of staff and the consequent degree of productivity depends. Staffing predictions and appointments of clinical leaders must assure that the education of the staff for their particular levels of responsibilities is provided and that the staff is melded into a group which is goal-directed toward quality patient care. A staff cannot meet the requirements for care if they are not prepared to do so. Preservice education alone does not assure that an adequate base is present for high quality functioning.

HOW ARE STAFFING PATTERNS PREDICTED?

The application of the classification schemes to projection of workload requires the computation of the amount of time required for the "average" patient in each class and the nursing care knowledge and skill level for each class of patients. The calculation of the number of nursing hours required for the average patient in each class per 24 hours is the first step in staffing predictions. Next, following determination of what comprises an "average group" of patients on the nursing unit, one derives the total number of nursing care hours per day per nursing unit. The distribution of the total hours required for an average group of patients on the nursing unit among both professional and nonprofessional staff follows. The ratio between the various categories of workers has been approached through task analysis, compilation of task complexes, and use of judgment by the nurse most knowledgeable about the nursing care of the patients to be served. No wholly defensible method is employed. However, the establishment of a ratio supposedly provides the "mix" of knowledge and skill required. After the mix has been determined, the distribution of hours of nursing personnel in the various categories over 24 hours is made by setting up specific numbers of staff for the day, evening, and night period. This distribution is used in the staffing pattern, which is defined as the work schedule for employees and which denotes on-duty time as well as days off.

Construction of an acceptable staffing pattern must take into account the policy regarding registered nurse supervision and direction at all times; the optimization of workload and supply of nurse personnel power; guidelines for personnel scheduling (policies regarding vacation, number of consecutive work days, minimum time lapse between scheduled tours of duty and work week); the various definitions of different nursing functions; and appropriate utilization of nursing knowledge and skill held by the workers in the different categories.

The records of the nursing department should contain documentation of the staffing determinations. Various types of forms are available in the literature for use as models for data collection. The purpose in using forms must be recognized. To collect data in an unrelated system without giving thought to how it will be used is the approach of the inexperienced. An accumulation of facts, without purpose, requires endless time and storage space.

HOW DOES ONE EVALUATE THE ADEQUACY OF A STAFFING PREDICTION?

Often staffing predictions are made, but an appraisal of their adequacy is never made. The ultimate test of a staffing program, or any nursing activity, is its effect upon the patient. The determination of effect upon patients requires criteria of care.

Developing criteria is time consuming and often imprecise. In the meantime, many nursing services are using a different approach to measurement of nursing quality related to nurse staffing. The use of this approach is referred to in the literature describing quality control systems and the nursing audit. Both of these topics entail the development of statements about the presence of attributes which are thought to be related to quality. These statements, for the most part, are concerned with the presence of conditions that are more likely to give rise to quality than to specific observations about the patient and his state. Other types of standards have arisen from the study of nursing tasks and are called time standards.

The ideal standards are those derived from analysis of patient outcomes and include specific positive statements about the change or condition observed in the patient or in the patient's environment as assurance that his condition can be maintained.

If we are going to measure the adequacy of our predictions for staffing, we must operationally define the appraisal of that adequacy. This appraisal requires deciding how to measure effect in the patient, how to quantify these results, and how to relate these data to numbers of staff and their cost. In making these decisions our major concern must be a statement of realistic and significant effects desired in the patient population served. These criteria are directly related, therefore, to objectives established for patients in the unit. This returns us to the first question asked, "What is the quality of the product to be delivered? What is its purpose?"

Although the quality of care provided and staffing have long been recognized as related, unfortunately, only a few studies examine the nature of that relationship. At the present time, few directors of nursing services have collected baseline data about either quality of care or staffing on nursing units which can serve as a basis for making judgments about the result of staff changes. Furthermore, the confounding effect of supervisory differences, individual variations in staff knowledge and skill, clinical variations of patient requirements, and other related variables make precise statements about the relation between amount of staff and quality of care impossible. Judgment about the need for an increase or decrease in staff is more reliable if it is based upon factual data about amount, qualifications, and combinations of nursing staff. The complex question, "How much staff and of what kind is required for high quality care?" cannot be answered until we address ourselves to these matters.

It is the purpose of the second part of Standard I of the Joint Commission on Hospital Accreditation to stimulate us into thinking about and acting on methods of quality measurement. Its intent is also to focus our attention on staffing, not as a mathematical exercise, but as a program of the department which has a broad conceptual base.

The success of staffing is always dependent upon the manpower provided, its intellectual quality and skills, the wise utilization of their talents in appropriate numbers and combinations, and their motivation to provide high quality. Clinical nursing leadership is the vital force in the movement toward staffing for high quality care.

REFERENCES

1. *Accreditation Manual for Hospitals 1970.* Chicago, Ill., Joint Commission on Accreditation of Hospitals, p. 49.
2. Aydelotte, M. K. *Survey of Nursing Services.* New York: National League for Nursing, 1968, p. 13.
3. Moore, M. A. Philosophy, Purpose and Objectives: Why Do We Have Them? *J. Nurs. Adm.* 1:9, 1971.

SOME MANAGEMENT TECHNIQUES FOR NURSING SERVICE ADMINISTRATORS

BY MARY ELLEN WARSTLER

Mary Ellen Warstler, R.N., M.A., who selected the articles to appear in this book, was Director of Nursing Service, Mercy Hospital, Springfield, Mass., when this article was written. The article is reprinted from JONA, November-December 1972. Ms. Warstler is now Director, Department of Nursing Services, American Nurses' Association.

The nursing service administrator along with the hospital administrator is being pressured by the consumers and payees of health care to justify the need for personnel and materials within economic and effective limitations. No longer can our reasons be based on opinions; they must be documented data in order to be convincing. The means described here are an attempt to meet this challenge to all hospitals.

Note: Credit is due the nursing staffs in the following hospitals where I have served as nursing service administrator for their valuable help in developing the forms and definitions discussed in this article: Research Hospital and Medical Center, Kansas City, Missouri; Maimonides Medical Center, Brooklyn, New York; St. Catherine's Hospital, East Chicago, Illinois; St. Ann's Hospital, Chicago, Illinois; Alexandria Hospital, Alexandria, Virginia; Mercy Hospital, Springfield, Massachusetts.

With an ever increasing awareness of the hospital as a major business, nursing service administrators have found a need for information to aid them in daily and long-term planning. Such aids must not only provide data on quantity needs, but must at the same time demonstrate a desirable level of quality care of patients.[1,2] Because the cost factors involved in obtaining quality care have become exorbitant, it is only natural that consumers and third party payors, including the government, require data to support hospital management within the limits of economic and effective use of both personnel and materials.

Most nursing service administrators are well aware of the pressures for supportive documentation and are looking for information on how best to develop techniques for obtaining the data necessary for such documentation. These data must cover a sufficiently long period of time to indicate cyclic changes and fluctuations. Changes or fluctuations may be, and often are, due to some or all of the following factors:

1. Patient occupancy percentages and their fluctuation month to month
2. Type and level of nursing needs of patients admitted for care
3. Age and physical dependency of patients
4. Types of complications suffered by patients
5. Frequency of rehospitalization
6. Relationship between maximum utilization of professional nursing personnel with paranursing personnel
7. Availability of personnel at periods of greatest need
8. Actual distribution of task activities, by time of day as well as by whom assigned
9. Continuity in available personnel and materials 7 days per week and 24 hours per day
10. Evidences of quality care of lack of same
11. Salaries
12. Cost of materials
13. Specific hospital situations

As yet our techniques for gathering some of this information are crude at best. The importance of finding ways to utilize these data, however, is of the highest order if nursing service administrators are to manage nursing services well and thus avoid capitulating to the outside influences, discussed above, that attempt to determine what the hospital and its nursing service can or should do.

At all times there is a great need for a high degree of clinical nursing competence on the part of both professional and paraprofessional nurses. Without a high quality of clinical nursing performance the management techniques discussed here are worthless. At the same time, without good nursing service management, high quality clinical nursing performance is often frustrated and prevents competent nurses from providing what is best for their patients. Without a willingness to test and apply knowledge gained from the fields of science and technology, nursing management cannot facilitate the delivery of quality care to patients.

The following group of management techniques in one way or another have a common dependency in the stage of collection or interpretation. Through illustrations and discussion I will try to demonstrate how these techniques can be adapted for use in the nursing service department of a hospital.

DEFINITIONS OF THE NURSING CARE NEEDS OF PATIENTS

Before personnel and materials necessary for nursing service can be determined it seems axiomatic that there be factual knowledge of the various types and degrees of nursing care needs in a given hospital setting. The first step,

therefore, is to define the categories of patients and their nursing needs.

The literature describes three different categories: Minimal (self), Intermediate, and Intensive.[3,4] At this time there seems to be no completely satisfactory system of categorizing patients according to care needs. In attempting to use the three-category system in five different hospitals, I have found it necessary to subdivide this system into five categories which reflect more nearly the specific needs of patients. Each group of nurses with whom I worked particularly found the intermediate category[5] too broad for dealing accurately with the various patient care needs when the categories were used to determine quantity of staff. Therefore this category was divided into minimal and intermediate care needs. Some of the same nurses also had problems in using the category of Intensive Care without dividing it into subcategories, one indicating patients who should be under the supervision of the intensive care or coronary care units and the other denoting patients considered very ill and in need of care just short of the high degree of care provided in the special care units. This division in some of the hospitals was in part necessary because patients normally considered as belonging in special care units were not always moved there by the physician, or the space in the special units was not sufficient to accommodate them, or no special unit had been established. Therefore requirements for nursing care on the general care units became much higher.

Such a distinction has merit when one realizes that for a patient requiring intensive care the average hours of nursing care in a 24-hour period is 10 to 14 hours and occasionally higher, whereas a patient considered quite ill in relation to convalescing patients requires only 7 to 8 hours of nursing care per 24 hours.

Table 1 describes the five categories, their titles, and a summary of the most common definitions.[6] In the five patient categories the definitions used are common for general adult medical and surgical patients. A separate set of definitions (Table 1) must be established for pediatric, maternity, newborn, and psychiatric patients. Definitions are needed for all other patients that do not quite fit into those indicated above. For teaching staff, the development of an extended set of specific examples of patients and their care needs has been helpful for each category and definition. These examples illustrate each category so that the data collected will be less a matter of personal opinion than might otherwise result with general definitions.

The data compiled from the daily record of patient care needs, as classified in the five-category system, can become the base for determining year round staffing needs for the annual hospital budget. I have found that this type of data is the best to present for justifying expenditures, especially when seeking additional staff because of changing needs. Such data would be equally effective when hospital and

TABLE 1

CATEGORIES OF NURSING CARE NEEDS OF PATIENTS

Category	Medical and Surgical (Adult and child) Patient	Maternity Patient	Newborn Infant	Psychiatric Patient
V Intensive Care	1. Acutely ill; requires constant or frequent observation; not necessarily terminal 2. Activity must be rigidly controlled 3. Requires continuous or very frequent treatment	1. Active antepartum or postpartum hemorrhage 2. Uncontrolled diabetic; eclampsia or severe pre-eclampsia; other severe medical problems 3. Premature labor; alcohol by·IV or other complications	1. Infants in isolettes for prematurity and requiring monitoring of O_2, IVs, apnea, etc. 2. Full-term infant who requires above care in an isolette	1. Acutely ill mentally and physically and requiring constant attention 2. Any new patient for first 24 hours
IV Modified intensive care	1. Acutely ill; requires frequent observation; may or may not be a terminal case 2. Limited activity; is dependant on others for basic needs 3. Requires frequent treatments	1. Acute or uncontrolled symptoms now under control 2. Cesarean section; for 24 hours PO 3. Postpartum first 12 hours 4. Threatened or incomplete abortion 5. Recovery room or labor room patients	1. Any newborn for first 24 hours 2. Babies in isolettes for observation for infection	1. Receiving IVs or requiring frequent observation or treatments 2. Motivation is limited; needs frequent supervision in ADL
III Intermediate care	1. Extreme symptoms have subsided or have not yet appeared; usually moderately ill 2. Behavior pattern deviates moderately yet does not require close observation 3. Activity must be partially controlled; or requires periodic treatment	1. Cesarean section; PO 24-72 hours 2. Postpartum 12-36 hours 3. Medical complication has been resolved	1. Any newborn after 24 hours who has stabilized body functions 2. Prematures in Armstrong heater or open crib until weight appropriate for discharge 3. Babies is isolette for phototherapy	1. Behavior pattern deviates moderately; requires moderate control of activity 2. Requires only periodic observation and treatment
II Minimal care	1. Mildly ill or convalescent 2. Activity is controlled requiring little treatment or observation 3. Needs very little help with personal hygiene	1. Requires only limited nursing observation or treatments		1. Awaiting discharge or transfer 2. Needing only slight control or little or no treatment

Category	Medical and Surgical (Adult and child) Patient	Maternity Patient	Newborn Infant	Psychiatric Patient
I Self-care	1. Usually ambulatory; activities are not limited; requires a minimum of observation 2. In hospital for x-rays and/or treatment or physical therapy	1. Awaiting x-ray or lab results, ready for discharge 2. Requires no personal care; able to have free activity		
O Special condition	Patients having one or more of the following conditions shall be classified as above but at one higher step of nursing care need. 1. Isolation for communicable or infectious disease 2. Handicap (blind, deaf, dumb, amputee) 3. Senility, confusion, or general debility of age 4. Incontinent or semicomatose or paraplegic 5. Continuous temperature above 102° or nonstable blood pressure			

nursing service administrators are asked to justify their particular patient care costs in relation to another hospital in the community or to all hospitals in a common geographic area.

Once the patient category definitions have been established, the next step is for the team leader or charge nurse to evaluate the nursing care needs of her patients each 8 hours. This information becomes the data recorded in the upper left corner of the "24-Hour General Patient Unit Report" (Table 2a). In order to make this procedure of reporting as simple as possible the following colored signals have been used in the nursing care Kardex:

Category V (Intensive care), red signal
Category IV (Modified intensive care), orange signal
Category III (Intermediate care), brown signal
Category II (Minimal care), blue signal
Category I (Self-care), green signal

In some cases we have introduced the use of a black signal to indicate that the critically ill Catholic patient has been anointed.

GENERAL PATIENT UNIT 24-HOUR REPORT

The 24-hour general patient report (Tables 2a, b, and c) is prepared by the unit clerical staff in cooperation with the team leader or charge nurse. It is actually a cumulative report representing the three work shifts (day, evening, and night). It serves to keep the area department heads (supervisors) and supervisors on the evening and night shifts in-

formed of important unit activity. It also lessens the length of the verbal report between shifts, whether done in person or by means of a tape recorder.

The general report from a specific unit is initiated by the day staff and added to by both evening and night personnel. It is submitted to the nursing service office an hour and a half before the end of each shift. This is necessary so that the data on available nursing personnel can be used for determining the needs for and assignment of float personnel before the next shift reports for work.

Directions given to the team leader or charge nurse who prepares or oversees the preparation of the 24-hour report are as follows:

1. The report is due in the nursing service office at 2:00 A.M., 10:00 P.M., and 5:00 A.M.
2. Check in red beside the name of any new admission if the patient is an employee or prominent person in the community.
3. Under the heading Preoperative Patients check if the history and physical examination have been taken and/or written, and if consent for the surgical procedure has been signed properly.
4. Under the heading Decubiti write in red at the time of admission if the patient was admitted with decubiti and indicate the location of same when reporting.
5. Briefly explain each unusual patient incident or accident which may have occurred, in addition to preparing written incident report.
6. Report on reverse side of sheet any unusual or negative progress of patients.

TABLE 2-A

MERCY HOSPITAL — SPRINGFIELD, MASS. 01104

GENERAL PATIENT UNIT—24 HOUR REPORT

Unit _____   Date _____

Census	I	II	III	IV	V	T	Rm #	Admitted Patient	Doctor	Time	Diagnosis - Remarks (Inc. VIP's - Emp.)	Admission Condition
2 pm												
10 pm												
5 am												

Isolation (Rms. & Diagnosis)

Rm	Name	Doctor	Diagnosis

Private Duty

Hr.	Rn	LPN	S
2p			
10p			
5p			

Vacant Rooms

Discharged

Rm #	Time

Pre-operative Patients

Rm	Patient	Doctor	P.O. Order	H/P	OR consent

Transferred

From	To

DECUBITI

Rm.	Name	Doctor	Condition

DEATHS

Rm.	Name	Doctor	Time	Autopsy

ERT'S

Rm.	Name	Doctor	Time	Condition

Incidents - Employee, Pt. Error, Theft, Med.

Feed Patients (Bed#)

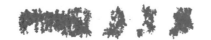

TABLE 2-B

PATIENT'S CONDITION

(Include only those who are not progressing well)

Rm.	Name	Doctor Diagnosis	7-3:30	3-11:30	11-7

Charge Nurse: Charge Nurse: Charge Nurse:

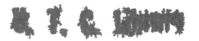

TABLE 2-C

SPECIAL AREA 24 HOUR REPORT

Report total number of patients handled in each **respective** shift and twenty-four hour total.

CASES	DAY	EVE	NITE	TOTAL
MAJOR O.R.				
E ENT O.R.				
MAJOR R.R.				
E ENT R.R.				
3W EXAM RM				
EMERGENCY RM				
CAST RM				
CLINIC (O.P.D.)				

General Summary of Incidents Related to Patients

_____

_____

_____

_____

_____

_____

_____

_____

_____

_____

_____

_____

_____

CHARGE NURSE

2 pm _____

10 pm _____

5 am _____

For those patient care areas using the 24-hour report (see Table 2c) it is returned each morning to the particular unit where it is filed for about 30 days for reference when needed. A few of the uses may be: (1) For the head nurse and/or team leader who has been on days off to know what occurred of significance regarding their patients. (2) For part-time nurses to obtain a quick review of the unit activity since last working day, or as background if a new assignment. (3) For general information, often requested by other departments, such as when patients were transferred and where, or discharged and to whom. (4) The interested head nurse can use it in providing some specific accumulative data about her unit for study and comparison.

The night assistant director of nursing service and staff summarizes the individual reports daily, after 5 A.M., into a Nursing Service Summary Report (Table 3) and delivers a copy to the director of nursing and the hospital administrator each morning. This summary report is filed in the nursing service office for a minimum of 31 days, or until all data for the following monthly reports have been recorded:

1. Infection Incident Report (by unit and total service)
2. Decubiti Incident Report (by unit and total service)
3. Daily census by categories for each unit
4. Other studies as indicated by interest or need

Other incidents and accidents are not summarized from this report (Table 3) as each is reported in written detail. These written reports are used to summarize the monthly incident and accident report.

At the end of each month, when the various reports are completed, a copy of each summary is distributed to each department head (supervisor) and head nurse. This has interested a number of unit personnel in improving their unit record of nursing care when the infection, decubiti, or incident reports have been unsatisfactory. The monthly report of daily census by categories has provided the department head and head nurse one means for studying nursing care needs as they relate to either the actual costs or with similar patient care units.

Annually these monthly reports are summarized and compared with past annual summaries. This review of comparative data from year to year provides a descriptive picture of nursing service needs and activities in the most factual manner known to me at this time. These data are also valuable supportive evidence when developing annual budgetary requests.

DAILY NURSING CARE HOURS DETERMINED FOR EACH UNIT

Once the categories of patient nursing care needs and the specific definitions have been established, it is possible to determine the total personnel hours required during each 24-hour period for each category. Over the past 12 years of comparative experiences, by means of the five-category system described I have been able to determine that the average and variations of personnel hours per patient per category are as follows:

Category V: Intensive care, usually requires 10 to 14 hours (average 12 hours)*
Category IV: Modified intensive care, usually requires 7 to 8 hours (average 7.5 hours)
Category III: Intermediate care, usually requires 5 to 6 hours (average 5.5 hours)
Category II: Minimal care, usually requires 3 to 4 hours (average 3.5 hours)
Category I: Self-care, usually requires 1 to 2 hours (average 1.5 hours)

This standard varies according to the physical arrangements of the patient care units and whether the greater amount of non-nursing activities for housekeeping, transportation, messenger, and mail service has been transferred outside the nursing service division.

With such standards one can quickly determine the number of nursing care hours needed versus the available nursing care hours on any specific day or for any specific period of time (Table 4). Once the *Daily Staffing* report is completed the person responsible for the daily staffing of patient care units can use the data in the columns headed Persons Over and Persons Under for distributing the available float staff or requesting relief from units with excess hours for the units lacking in available hours of personnel.

The data collected under the columns headed Total Students and Trainees become background information for deciding which unit has the greatest need for additional supportive personnel or which unit can spare some personnel for another unit. At no time are students or trainees considered working personnel. Since whatever learning experience each is having does affect the remaining workload it can be a useful factor for consideration when the nursing care needs are higher than available employed personnel. Our instructors (for both students and trainees, including new employees) weekly provide the person in charge of staffing with a schedule noting what these workers will be doing within each patient unit and the actual hours on the unit. At no time do we use either group for service over and above that contributed by the learning experience.

A research of accumulated daily hours of personnel needed versus the hours of personnel available (excluding students and trainees) is kept for the total nursing service and used as an indicator for budget adjustments and justification for future budget planning.

I have not yet been able to devise a satisfactory means for determining the proportion of needed hours of nursing care by various categories of nursing personnel, such as registered professional nurses, licensed practical nurses, and nurse aides (Table 1). This kind of information would be most helpful in evaluating whether the needed knowledges and skills are available for quality nursing care.

*The hours at the high end of the scale are appropriate to an institution in which few non-nursing duties have been re-assigned to non-nursing personnel. The lower range of hours may be appropriate to an institution in which there is a well functioning unit manager system.

TABLE 3

MERCY HOSPITAL
SUMMARY 24 HOUR REPORT, NURSING SERVICE

Date: _____ Signature _____

Census: _____ (5 a.m.)

Units	I	II	III	IV	V	T	Avail. Beds	CRITICAL PATIENTS				
								Rm	Name	Doctor	Diagnosis	Comment
TCU - gen.												
O.P.												
1W - gen.												
Psych.						╳	╳					
EST's						╳	╳					
2W												
2G												
3W												
4W - gen												
- Neuro.						╳	╳	VIP's & EMPLOYEES				
St.M								Rm	Name	Doctor	Diagnosis	Comment
Rehab.												
Ped. up 2 yr.												
2 - 6 yr.						╳	╳					
over 6 yr.						╳	╳					
O.P.								ALL INCIDENTS				
1CU ^{2} M								Brief description (Include Med. errors & thefts)				
S						╳	╳					
1CU ^{3} CC												
M						╳	╳					
	2		10		5	T		CARDIAC ARRESTS				
3W. Exam								Rm	Name	Doctor	Time	Cond.
Major OR												
EENT OR												
Major Rec.												
EENT Rec.												

DECUBITI

RM	Name	Doctor	Area	Condition

DEATHS

Rm	Name	Doctor	Time	Autopsy

ISOLATION

Rm	Name	Doctor	Diag.	Cond

Feeds: (area & #)

TABLE 4

MERCY HOSPITAL
Nursing Service

DAILY STAFFING

NURSING DIVISION

DATE:

AREA	PATIENT ACUITY CENSUS										CENSUS	Total Hours Needed *	TOTAL PERSONS NEEDED	Persons Needed			Persons Available			Persons Over			Persons Under			Total Stud.			Trainees			
	Cl I PTS	1.5 HRS	Cl II PTS	3.5 HRS	Cl III PTS	5.5 HRS	Cl IV PTS	7.5 HRS	Cl V PTS	12 HRS				DAY 47%	EVE 35%	NITE 17%	D	E	N	D	E	N	D	E	N	SN	PN	T	RN	LPN	NA	CK

TOTAL
AVERAGE HRS. PER PT. DAY NEEDED.

TOTAL
AVER. HRS. PER PT. DAY AVAILABLE

TOTAL COL 1, 2, 3
AVER. HRS. PER PT. DAY GRAND TOTAL

TOTAL
AVER. HRS. PER PT. DAY

(STUDENTS) (TRAINEES)

* Total Nsg hours need ÷ 7.5 = Total persons needed

REFERENCES

1. Saren, M., and Straub, A. Nursing Service Effectiveness, *Hospitals, J.A.H.A.* 44(2): 45, 1970.
2. Young, J. P. A Method for Allocation of Nursing Personnel to Meet Inpatient Care Needs. A component study under U.S. Public Health Service Research Grant GN-5537, Operations Research Division, Baltimore: The Johns Hopkins Hospital, 1962.
3. Connor, R. J., Flagle, C. D., Hoeih, R. K. C., Preston, R. A., and Singer, S. Effective Use of Nursing Resources—A Research Report, *Hospitals, J.A.H.A.* 35(9): 5, 1961.
4. McCartney, R. A., McKee, B., and Cady, L. D. Nurse Staffing Systems, *Hospitals, J.A.H.A.* 44(22): 102, 1970.
5. Clark, E. L., R. N., and Dibbs, W. W. Quantifying Patient Care Needs. *Hospitals, J.A.H.A.* 45(18): 96, 1971.

Cyclic Work Schedules
and
a Nonnurse Coordinator
of Staffing

by Mary Ellen Warstler

Ms. Warstler is also the author of the preceding article and her biographic data appears there. This article is reprinted from JONA, November-December 1973.

Cyclic staffing, providing every other weekend off for nursing service employees, is described as an attempt to supply full hospital care seven days per week. A nonnurse coordinator of the staffing plan is used in place of the professional nurse supervisor to prepare the weekly work schedules. This arrangement enables professional nurses to spend more time in patient care supervision and staff development activities.

Many hospitals are making the effort to fully utilize their facilities seven days a week. The success of the effort is contingent upon achieving balanced staffing each day of the week to meet the patient care needs. Yet there is an ever-increasing demand by staff for every other weekend off. In hospitals where every other weekend off is policy, the most frequent complaint from nursing supervisors and general staff is the shortage of weekend personnel.

Few hospitals are able to provide good, safe care for patients on weekends with only fifty percent of the regular staff on duty. The solution for this weekend dilemma requires a great deal of prior planning which can be achieved by establishing cyclic work schedules. Once the proper schedule has been worked out, it becomes possible for a nonnurse coordinator of staffing to maintain the program with a minimum of supervision by professional nursing personnel. In institutions with computer services, many aspects of such a program can be readily computerized, adding another time-saving factor to a presently time-consuming job, whether performed by a nurse or a nonnurse employee.

The management techniques for nursing service administrators to be discussed are confined to the development of a workable cyclic schedule and the use of a nonnurse coordinator for daily staffing in the central nursing service office. How the cyclic schedule simplifies preparation of the weekly assignment sheet of working hours for each patient care unit and how daily readjustments can be made in the distribution of personnel to meet the daily fluctuations in care needs of patients are the basis for the discussion.

PREPLANNING PREPARATION FOR CYCLIC STAFFING PROGRAM

It is necessary to have available the classification of patients according to their nursing care needs and the determined number of nursing care hours required for each 24-hour period in order to establish manpower needs for the nursing service. Not considered, due to lack of documented data, is the proportion of the determined hours needed for each classification that must be contributed by professional, technical, and auxiliary nursing personnel if the desired level of quality care is to be achieved. Such information combined with the classification system and total personnel hours for each hospital would complete the necessary model, as defined by Berkeley [1], to justify variable manpower needs among health care institutions.

The categories of patients and nursing care hours needed are referred to throughout this article. The definitions and discussion of the determination of the nursing care hours were discussed in detail in earlier article [2]. The development and use of the following categories and required staffing hours discussed in that article were limited to use in short-term, acute care hospitals varying in size from 225 to 400 beds and are as follows:

Category I: *Self-care* usually requires 1 to 2 hours, with an average of 1.5 hours per 24 hours.

Category II: *Minimal care* usually requires 3 to 4 hours, with an average of 3.5 hours per 24 hours.

Category III: *Intermediate care* usually requires 5 to 6 hours, with an average of 5.5 hours per 24 hours.

Category IV: *Modified intensive care* usually requires 7 to 8 hours, with an average of 7.5 hours per 24 hours.

Category V: *Intensive care* usually requires 10 to 14 hours, with an average of 12 hours per 24 hours.

It is necessary to keep a record by individual patient unit as to the daily and monthly average distribution of the daily census by the number of patients within each patient classification as to needed nursing care. Such a record becomes the basis for projecting the maximum, average, and minimum levels of daily hours of personnel needed by an individual unit. The total computation of this data for all patient units becomes a basis for the number of personnel needed each day to maintain a sufficient number of man hours to meet the nursing care needs of a particular hospital.

Once the daily man hours are determined for a particular hospital, it is then necessary to convert this total into the hours needed annually. Before a final man hour budget proposal can be made, it is necessary to determine the vacation and holiday needs of each person working on a permanent basis. Adjustments must be made for replacement of anticipated paid absences. The accumulated man hours from this total data then becomes the basis for the proposed budget.

Upon approval of a budget the next step is to establish the nursing service position control for each patient unit (Table 1) so that it serves as a measure of control for the approved budgeted man hours. Thereafter any revisions of this position control should be supported by the accumulated data from the classification of patients in categories of nursing care needs. The most unreliable aspect of the nursing service position control illustrated is that of determining the number of positions to be allocated among professional, technical, and auxiliary personnel. Without documented data as a model, the best available assistance in determining the levels of personnel needs are the opinions of head nurses and professional staff along with other limited indicators within a particular institution.

Usually the approved man hour budget is based on a near average need for total personnel to meet total nursing care needs throughout the hospital. Everyone is acutely aware of the periods when a unit has a maximum need for personnel above the regular staff. However, studies indicate that there are usually units during the same period with underutilization of personnel due to minimum nursing care needs. Therefore, personnel from the units having underutilization of personnel can assist the units having overutilization of personnel and thus provide nearly balanced staffing within the same budget plan. These studies showed that when approximately fifteen percent of total manpower hours from each unit were assigned to a floating group, the daily varying manpower needs between units were utilized in a more efficient manner [3]. Experience in certain institutions support these findings [4]. It is advis-

TABLE I **Nursing Service Position Control**						
Area 2 West			Fund 811		Capacity 25	Average Census (last Year) 23
No.	Category	Hr	Shift	Cycle	Name	Remarks
A	Dept. Head	12	D	— —	A. Hogen	
1	Head Nse.	40	D	2	C. Suma	
1R	RN, TL	16	D	2R	H. Wong	
2	RN, TL	40	D	3	H. Evers, 24 hr	
					F. Collins, 16 hr	
2R	RN, TL	16	D	3R	K. Henry	
4	NA	40	D	5	S. Daniels	Expect repl. 10/8
4R	NA	16	D	5R	D. White	Works every weekend
7	WD, CK	40	D	8	M. Strand	
7R	WD, CK	16	D	8R	A. Smith	
9	RN, TL	40	E	10	S. Adams, 24 hr	Head Nurse will provide weekly work
9R	RN, TL	16	E	10R	M. Dowling, 16 hr	schedule
					Z. Walton, 16 hr	
10	LPN	40	E	11	W. Gripe	
10R	LPN	16	E	11R	T. Standish	
11	NA	40	E	12	E. Michaels	due out of orient. 10/15
11R	NA	16	E	12R	L. Marx	
12	WD, CK	40	E	13	C. Apple	
12R	WD, CK	40	E	13R	R. Strong	
13	RN, TL	40	N	13	P. Dixon	Wants W & Th, F & Sa off for cycle
13R	RN, TL	16	N	13R	S. Josephson	Will work W & Th, F & Sa
14	LPN	40	N	14	M. Trumball	
14R	LPN	16	N	14R	M. Wald	

able to assign personnel in this special float group to the same units as much as possible or within units having similar kinds of patients assigned, e.g., medicine, surgery, and obstetrics, so that each employee becomes well oriented to the nursing care needs and physical facilities of units to which they will be most frequently assigned.

DEVELOPMENT OF A SPECIFIC CYCLIC PLAN

The cyclic staffing program and its various advantages have been described in many articles [5,6]. It seems wise, however, to emphasize a few of these advantages:

1. Days off for personnel are known so that social plans and family responsibilities can be planned in advance.

2. A controlled maximum number of work periods before a day off is provided.

3. A nearly balanced number of personnel on duty each day and shift is facilitated.

4. The ability to use part-time personnel when and where needed rather than the costly practice of hiring additional full-time personnel, needed or not, results in cost savings.

The particular cyclic staffing plan to be used by a nursing service depends on (1) the frequency of free weekends for personnel, (2) the policy on the maximum number of working periods before a day off or rest period, (3) provisions for part-time relief personnel, (4) variations in the work load on different days of the week, and (5) whether or not inservice programs are planned on a day when all personnel will be on duty.

The particular cyclic staffing program to be described (Table 2) was based on the policies of (1) every other weekend off for all personnel, (2) a weekly or biweekly pay period, (3) commonly a maximum of five days of work before a rest period, (4) permanent evening and night personnel except in emergencies due to unavoidable absences or vacancies, (5) equal staffing man hours seven days a week, (6) permanent relief personnel scheduled within a particular patient unit so that there would always be some full-time personnel on duty to assure continuity of care plans.

To maintain equal man hours of duty for every day of the week it was necessary to plan for one relief person to work 16 hours a week for each 40-hour position. When all personnel worked a 40-hour week it was impossible to eliminate overlapping days of work and meet the policy for every other weekend off.

The cyclic work schedule in Table 2 is based on a 10-week period which continuously repeats itself. Before the cyclic pattern was applied to the nursing service position control (Table 1) the approved man hours were first divided into 56-hour components and each component was divided into a position of 40 hours for the full-time staff person, and 16 hours for the part-time staff person. In cases in which the approved man hours could not be

divided into equal components, the few excess hours were added to the temporary personnel reserve to meet emergency needs in addition to the regular float staff.

Each full-time, 40-hour person was assigned to one of the ten cyclic patterns (Table 2). The part-time person assigned to complete the 56-hour component was assigned the same cyclic pattern number, with the letter "R" added to indicate that the person was to be the relief. For example, the 40-hour person was assigned cycle number 8, and the 16-hour person was assigned cycle 8R (Table 3). In assigning specific numbers, every other head nurse was assigned to cycle 1 or cycle 2 in order to assure that fifty percent of the head nurse staff was on duty at any one time. This same pattern was followed on the evening and night shifts so that at all times fifty percent of the full-time assistant head nurse staff was on duty. On each of the three shifts the rest of the personnel positions on the specific shifts were assigned sequential numbers. In this way there was maintained a continuity of staff with knowledge of the patient care needs and full-time personnel in sufficient numbers to support part-time personnel at all times (Table 1).

Once the cyclic pattern was established and all positions were assigned a number, new personnel were automatically assigned the number given the position before it became vacant. Persons desiring to transfer to different units or shifts had to change their schedule to conform to the schedule assigned to the position to which they were transferred. Otherwise the carefully established balance of the staffing would be upset. Even though this limitation

TABLE 2 **10 Week Cyclic Program**

Regular full-time employee's day off (X)							
	S	M	T	W	Th	F	S	Corresponds to
1st week		X					X	Week 1 of cycle 1
2nd week	X					X		Week 1 of cycle 2
3rd week		X					X	Week 1 of cycle 3
4th week	X				X			Week 1 of cycle 4
5th week			X				X	Week 1 of cycle 5
6th week	X					X		Week 1 of cycle 6
7th week				X			X	Week 1 of cycle 7
8th week	X				X			Week 1 of cycle 8
9th week		X					X	Week 1 of cycle 9
10th week	X			X				Week 1 of cycle 10

Regular part-time relief employee's work days (W)							
1st week		W					W	Week 1 of cycle 1R
2nd week	W					W		Week 1 of cycle 2R
3rd week		W					W	Week 1 of cycle 3R
4th week	W				W			Week 1 of cycle 4R
5th week			W				W	Week 1 of cycle 5R
6th week	W					W		Week 1 of cycle 6R
7th week				W			W	Week 1 of cycle 7R
8th week	W				W			Week 1 of cycle 8R
9th week		W					W	Week 1 of cycle 9R
10th week	W			W				Week 1 of cycle 10R

may appear difficult, in actual practice there are many ways to meet personnel needs within the boundaries of a balanced staffing program.

In situations in which institutions depend on a higher number of part-time nurses than alloted for in the position control (Table 1), and full-time nurses are unavailable, it is possible to fill a full-time position with available part-time personnel when combined working hours do not exceed a 40-hour week and conform to the days to be worked by the particular position. Occasionally two or three persons can satisfactorily combine their available time to cover seven continuous working days. This arrangement often will allow part-time personnel who cannot meet regular cyclic requirements to work permanently the days of their choice. Another common exception that allows the staff flexibility in meeting personal needs that may arise is to allow the full-time person and her relief to rearrange days off for a temporary period of time.

TEMPORARY PERSONNEL REGISTRY

For persons limited to specific working days and unable to meet the foregoing requirements, a register of temporary personnel who can be called on a day-by-day or week-by-week basis to fill vacancies and unexpected absences can be established. This kind of registry is extremely valuable in meeting nursing care needs on days when the nursing care factor is higher than usual, or during heavy vacation or illness periods. Personnel listed in the temporary register are allowed to specify the shift or part shift, the day of the week, and the patient unit in which they prefer to work. This differs from permanent personnel who must work full shifts and according to the cyclic schedule on their units.

PUTTING CYCLIC STAFFING PROGRAM INTO OPERATION

When all the preplanning for changeover to a cyclic work program has been completed and the effective date has been set, a series of meetings should be held so that each individual is able to hear about the new plans. Since readjustments for some staff are inevitable, there should be a period of time allowed before the effective date for working out a schedule of hours around the few personnel who find it impossible to adjust to the regular cyclic work schedule. The person handling these special problems of personnel, should be knowledgeable in the many possible adjustments within the framework of the plan as well as understand and be appreciative of individual personnel needs.

During general meetings each staff member should receive a copy of her assigned cyclic schedule for study and for adjustment of personal obligations where possible. It usually takes personnel about three months to adjust their personal time around the new hours. It is advisable that personnel be willing to make adjustments in hours during this transition period.

THE NONNURSE STAFFING COORDINATOR

Once the cyclic work schedules have been established, it is a simple matter for the nonnurse employee (either male or female) in the central nursing office to prepare the weekly work schedule for each unit. This weekly work schedule incorporates only the necessary adjustments weekly, which may have to be made either because of patient care needs or personal requests. On each Thursday, prior to the week it becomes effective, the weekly schedule for each unit is posted on the unit bulletin board and a copy is kept by the staffing coordinator. Daily, or as often as needed, the coordinator calls personnel who

TABLE 3 Your Personal Cyclic Schedule

Name of employee

Your day off cyclic schedule is # 8. Your beginning date of work is indicated at the week corresponding to the days off for your 1st week on duty. Thereafter follow each week's schedule in consecutive sequence. Anyone required to rotate from day to evenings or nights will have such hours made out by respective head nurse.

Date Cycle Begins	Week of Cycle	S	M	T	W	Th	F	Sa
	1	X				X		
	2			X				X
	3	X			X			
	4		X					X
	5	X					X	
	6		X					X
	7	X				X		
	8			X				X
	9	X					X	
	10				X			X

Your days to work cyclic schedule is # 8R. Your date of work is indicated at the week corresponding to the hours to be worked for your 1st. week on duty. Thereafter follow each week's schedule in consecutive sequence.

Date Cycle Begins	Week of Cycle	S	M	T	W	Th	F	Sa
	1	W				W		
	2			W				W
	3	W			W			
	4		W					W
	5	W					W	
	6		W					W
	7	W				W		
	8			W				W
	9	W					W	
	10				W			W

TABLE 4

Mercy Hospital Nursing Service Daily Staffing Chart

NURSING DIVISION

DATE

PATIENT ACUITY CENSUS

AREA	C1.I PTS.	1.5 HRS.	C1.II PTS.	3.5 HRS.	C1.III PTS.	5.5 HRS.	C1.IV PTS.	7.5 HRS.	C1.V PTS.	12 HRS.	CENSUS	Total Hours Needed ★	Total Persons Needed	Persons Needed DAY 47%	EVE 35%	NITE 17%	Persons Available D E N	Persons Over D E N	Persons Under D E N	Total Stud. SN PN T	Trainees RN LPN NA CK

TOTAL

AVERAGE HRS. PER PT. DAY NEEDED.

TOTAL

AVER. HRS. PER PT. DAY AVAILABLE

TOTAL

AVER. HRS. PER PT. DAY

TOTAL COL 1, 2, 3

AVER. HRS. PER PT. DAY GRAND TOTAL

(STUDENTS)   (TRAINEES)

*Total Nsg hours need ÷ 7.5 = Total persons needed

are on the temporary personnel registry to fill unexpected vacancies. Throughout the work week any absences, overtime, called-in personnel, or unexpected changes in days off are recorded on the copy of personnel time kept by the staffing coordinator. This copy then becomes a permanent record and is used in preparing the payroll.

The daily staffing form (Table 4) can be prepared anytime after all admissions for the day have been accomplished. It has been observed that data about the patient's nursing needs are most accurate when the night personnel compile it, following a 5 A.M. collection of patient care unit reports. In this way the night emergencies are included, many of which require a high ratio of nursing care hours. Table 5 has been established so that the person recording the information does not spend unnecessary time in routine calculations. The daily staffing form (Table 4) is placed on the coordinator's desk at 7:00 A.M. When the coordinator reports for duty, she first studies the patient acuity census distribution on the daily staffing form, noting which units are over- or understaffed. Before scheduling the unassigned staff reporting at 7:00 A.M., she refers to the number of nursing care hours to be contributed by either students or trainees (new employees) under supervision of the staff education department. When such nursing care hours total the equivalent of eight hours,* that unit is credited with the equivalent of an additional person. If the total hours are equivalent to less than one person, no numerical value in personnel hours is given this contribution to nursing care. If, however, the student and trainee equivalent is one person or more and the unit already has a surplus of personnel, the staff coordinator calls the head nurse and asks that the number of permanent nursing staff over those required be sent to a comparable unit in need. Such switching of personnel is rarely necessary if the unit has been staffed so that fifteen percent of the average needed staff is assigned into a pool of float personnel.

The coordinator next will distribute unassigned staff from float personnel to units short of man hours. She refers to information provided her by the area supervisor as to the capabilities of the persons being sent and whether they can meet specific needs. In her preparation for the job as coordinator she has been taught the meaning of various patient categories and the ratios of nursing care needed. She is therefore able to recognize quickly that a unit which needs more help because there is a large number of category IV or category V patients, or both, should have an additional RN, or that a unit with many category I and II patients can manage with additional help from nurse aides, or a unit high in category III patients can be helped best with LPNs, RNs, or both, depending on the staffing distribution already present on the particular unit.

*At Mercy Hospital student hours were credited as one-third of actual scheduled time on the unit while new employees were credited as one-half of actual scheduled time on the unit.

Unless the daily requests for replacements to fill vacancies are unduly high in number, the staffing coordinator can keep the master copy of nursing service positions (Table 1) up to date, inform the personnel department of all personnel changes, and maintain cumulative records for use in future planning.

Once she knows the job well, the staffing coordinator requires counseling by professional nursing personnel only for exceptional situations. Usually the experience has been that a nonnurse in this position frequently is able to get assistance from off duty persons in time of special need with more willingness than when the professional nurse, usually a supervisor, makes such calls.

The cyclic work schedule for staffing and the nonnurse staffing coordinator make it possible to relieve head nurses and supervisors of time-consuming clerical details, enabling them to spend more of their time in patient care supervision and direction. It also requires a smaller salary budget for the coordinating activity than when a professional nurse has to do the coordinating of the schedules instead of practicing nursing care or teaching, for which she was primarily educated.

TABLE 5 Pre-calculated Data for Completing Daily Staffing Chart

Calculation of Individuals Needed Each Shift				
Total Nursing Care Hours Needed	Total Persons ÷ 7.5	Day 47%	Evening 35%	Night 17%
64	9	4	3	2
71	10	5	4	2
86	12	6	4	2
94	13	6	5	2
101	14	7	5	
109	15	7		
117	16	8		
124	17			
133 etc.				

Calculation of Nursing Care Hours Needed					
Number of Patients	(1.5) C1	(3.5) C2	(5.5) C3	(7.5) C4	(12.0) C5
1	1.5	3.5	5.5	7.5	12.0
2	3.0	7.0	11.0	15.0	24.0
3	4.5	11.5	16.5	22.5	36.0
4	6.0	14.0	22.0	30.0	
5	7.5	17.5	27.5		
6	9.0	21.0	33.0		
7	10.5	24.5			
8	12.0				
9 etc.					

REFERENCES

1. Berkeley, E. C. Not understanding a computer. *Comput. Automat.* 20(2): 6, 1971.
2. Warstler, M. E. Management techniques for nursing service administrators. *JONA* 2(6): 26, 1972.
3. Connor, R. J., Fagle, C. D., Hsieh, R. K. C., Preston, R. A., and Singer, S. Effective use of nursing resources: A research report. *Hospitals J.A.H.A.* 35(9): 33, 1961.
4. Bauer, J. Clinical staffing with a 10-hour day work week. *JONA* 1(6): 12, 1971.
5. Bauer, J. Four-day workweek? Oh, those long weekends! *R.N.* 35(1): 42, 1972.
6. Morrish, A. R., and O'Connor, A. R. Cyclic scheduling *JONA* 1(5): 49, 1971.

SELECTED BIBLIOGRAPHY

Hilgar, E.   Unit management system. *JONA* 2(1): 43, 1972.

McCartney, R. A., McKee, B., and Cady, M. R.   Nurse staffing systems. *Hospitals, J.A.H.A.* 44(22): 102, 1970.

Paulson, V. M.   Nursing toward workable and humane solutions. *Hospitals, J.A.H.A.* 46(7): 143, 1972.

Connor, R. A. Work sampling study of variations in nursing work load. *Hospitals, J.A.H.A.* 35(9): 40, 1961.

Feyerherm, A. M., and Kirk, W. R.   Effect of census variation on nursing activity patterns. *Hospitals, J.A.H.A.* 38(8): 62, 1964.

The Reconstructed Work Week:

One Answer to the Scheduling Dilemma

by Lorraine P. Fraser

Restructure of the work week by altering the length of each shift and reducing the number of worked days at the same time, combined with a simple two-week schedule cycle that alternates work periods of reasonable length with adequate rest periods, has proved successful. This rearrangement of the work week makes even distribution of staff over the seven days of a week and fulfillment of employee expectations without additional cost.

Lorraine P. Fraser, R.N., M.A., is Director of Nursing, Jordan Hospital, Plymouth, Mass. The article is reprinted from JONA, September-October 1972.

Work schedules have been a major source of frustration for hospital nursing personnel for many years, and frequently they have been responsible for isolation of nurses from other members of society. As nursing has changed from a total life commitment to a profession combined with family life and/or other social commitments, the need to revise work schedules for nurses to coincide with current social patterns and expectations has become more pressing. Health care has become more complex, and the need for expert nursing care for the hospitalized patient knows no time limits. At the same time, hospitals, increasingly pressured by public concern, must limit expenses in order to curtail the spiraling cost of health care.

A large portion of the total hospital budget is allocated for nursing service labor costs; therefore an increase in these costs usually results in greater cost to the patient. In order to limit nursing service labor costs, directors of nursing must examine not only nursing care methodology and the types of services expected of nursing personnel but also scheduling practices and procedures. Under the traditional methods of scheduling the current expectations of nursing personnel cannot be met without incurring excess cost or accepting periods of inadequate staffing. Restructure of the work week is one way to provide adequate nursing care throughout each day, seven days per week, while providing, at the same time, a simple, predictable work schedule with stable work groups that reduces employee fatigue and enables nursing personnel to pursue other interests and activities.

The Scheduling Problem

When a work schedule for hospital nursing personnel must be planned within the traditional limits of an eight-hour day and a five-day week, there are several inherent problems involved. If a majority of the nursing personnel work full time, they must work two weekends of every three to make even distribution of personnel possible throughout the seven days of the week. In order to make it possible to recruit and retain nursing personnel, however, many hospitals have had to agree to give all nursing personnel every other weekend and holiday off. As a result, the hospital must choose between two basic alternative patterns of staffing in order to provide nursing care within reasonable budgetary limits.

One alternative is to hire as many full-time employees as possible and to accept the resultant understaffing on weekends or holidays and the overstaffing on some of the other days of the week. In addition, a nursing service that provides clinical experience for nursing students or other health care workers often finds the problem of overstaffing on weekdays further compounded. On some days of the week there may be two, three, or more times as many persons on duty as there are on other days. In this situation there is little chance to develop efficient and effective work patterns; consequently employees may develop a deep sense of frustration in their work. Absenteeism results in such situations as much from overstaffing as from understaffing. Some employees cannot tolerate the overstaffing or the "floating" that results from it. Other employees may not be able to face working on days when staffing is at its lowest level, usually Saturdays, Sundays, and holidays. The problems of excessive workloads and employee frustration are then further aggravated.

The available time on overstaffed days could well be used for inservice education, meetings, special assignments or projects, and the like, but few nursing services are able to plan adequately for these activities.

The second alternative is to limit the number of full-time employees and to hire one part-time employee to cover for each full-time employee. In order to keep the number of personnel on duty balanced seven days a week, the part-time employee would have to work only two days a week, including every other weekend. This choice provides equitable coverage more economically, but it may be impossible to hire enough part-time nursing personnel to accomplish this scheduling objective. An employee who is willing to work every other weekend usually insists on working more than one other day each week, and it is seldom possible to schedule additional days that coincide with the unplanned absence of other personnel. One extra day per week for each part-time employee is often accepted, a practice that results in an excess cost close to 15 percent of the minimum necessary for equitable coverage (one extra day per week for every seven days needed). In situations in which it is necessary for day personnel to rotate shifts, the full-time employee often has to work more evening and night shifts than would be necessary if part-time employees were required to rotate shifts in proportion to the number of hours worked or if all personnel worked full time and rotated.

Besides the problems outlined above, many married nurses with children cannot work an eight-hour shift and will work only if a shorter shift is available. When they are allowed to work a short evening shift, the full-time employees' day shift hours must be adjusted so that someone works until the part-time employee is available. Except in hospitals where a split shift is still used, this adjustment usually leads to less than adequate coverage during the first few hours of the day. Moreover, the nurses who work the short shift are often required to float—a distasteful practice that more often than not excludes them from patient care planning and makes effective supervision difficult, if not impossible.

Development of a New Work Schedule

For one general hospital, it became apparent that some of the basic scheduling problems could be resolved if the traditional limits of eight hours a day, five days a week were eliminated. Russell Moberly, a consultant who was working with the hospital on a wage and salary program, suggested that longer shifts with fewer work days per week be considered. Dr. Moberly knew of several industrial companies that had made similar changes successfully and he felt that the practice was spreading. At the time we considered changing the structure of the work week, there were twice as many part-time as full-time registered and practical nurses on the staff. Furthermore, the evening hours were covered primarily by part-time employees, most of whom worked fewer than eight hours per shift.

We considered the use of two twelve-hour shifts per day but ruled out this approach for several reasons. The number of employees on duty could not be balanced over the seven days of each week without using a basic schedule several weeks in length or incurring required overtime costs. In addition, state law limited the length of the work day for a female employee, and we felt it was desirable to work within this law rather than to challenge it. We also felt that few nurses would be willing or able to work a twelve-hour shift, and we were concerned about how effective a nurse might be toward the end of such a shift.

After considering the factors involved, we decided upon a short evening shift with two other shifts, each long enough so that a full-time employee who worked half of the days in each fourteen-day pay period would average 35 to 40 hours of work per week. We made the day shift 7 a.m. to 5 p.m., the night shift 9 p.m. to 7 a.m. and the evening shift 5 p.m. to 10 p.m. (see Fig. 1). By using these hours the employees on the night shift could still arrive home in time to get children off to school or to make the family car available for someone else's use. The day shift employees could be home for dinner at a reasonable hour, and the evening shift employees could get home at a more convenient hour without starting work much earlier than 6 p.m. as previously required. We wanted to overlap all shifts but decided against this because we felt that it would be extremely difficult to get enough personnel to cover on the night and evening shifts.

The basic work cycle chosen was two weeks long. Each employee would be scheduled to work Monday, Tuesday, Friday, and Saturday of one week and Sunday, Wednesday, and Thursday of the other week. Half of the employees would be scheduled for the first week of the cycle while the other half would be scheduled for the second week of the cycle (see Fig. 2). Under this work schedule each employee would have two consecutive days off in each week *plus* a three-day weekend every other week. At the same time, no work stretch would be longer than three days in succession.

Implementation of the New Work Schedule

Once we established the shifts and chose the basic schedule of days to be worked, two problems remained: (1) how to handle salaries and wages within the existing computerized payroll system and (2) how to implement, or at least test, the new work schedule.

After considering many ways of calculating employee compensation, we realized that an employee would receive

FIGURE 1

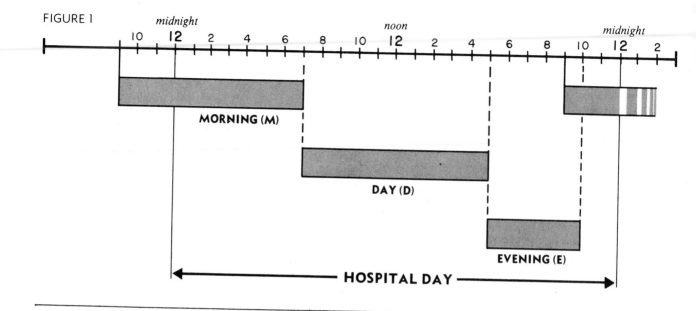

FIGURE 1

almost equivalent compensation each year if we continued most existing policies and payroll procedures. The only change needed was to discontinue the practice of giving an extra day off in each holiday week. This change posed no problem because the total number of hours actually worked per year already would be less than in the existing system. Furthermore, it would also have been impractical and costly to allow an extra day off for holidays because someone would be required to work an extra day in order to maintain the daily balance in personnel on duty.

We did, however, alter the basic schedule whenever necessary to assure each employee alternate holidays off. Because of the simplicity of the schedule, these adjustments could be planned and published far in advance (see Fig. 3).

Initially most nursing personnel, including supervisors, thought that we were unrealistic to think that anyone would work ten hours a day regularly. One head nurse, however, saw the potential benefits for herself and her family and wanted to try it. After many discussions with various groups, repeated requests for a volunteer group to try the schedule, and assurance that such volunteers would be allowed to return to the traditional schedule if they wished to do so after a trial of six to eight weeks, personnel slated to staff a new coronary care unit agreed to try the schedule when the unit opened.

After a delay of several months, the trial period for the new work schedule began. Not long afterwards one of the nurses assigned to the trial unit for a limited number of weeks began telling other employees that she might like to stay there because she liked the new work schedule. We quickly suggested that she could continue on this schedule and still return to her original unit if she could convince the other full-time nurses on that unit that they ought to try it too. Within three months, two other units had agreed to try the schedule. From then on we received requests for trial periods from individuals and small groups throughout the nursing service department. At first we insisted that *all* full-time employees on a given unit agree to try it as a group. Later we decided that this stipulation was not always necessary. Anyone who wanted to go on the new work schedule was allowed to do so as long as it would not increase the scheduling problems for the unit. In nine months, all ten inpatient units were using the schedule. (The operating room and the outpatient department were not included because their work load was not evenly spread over ten or more consecutive hours of each day.)

Implementation of the New Work Schedule for Unit Services Personnel

We had previously initiated a unit service program within the nursing service department. We knew that it would be necessary to provide adequate unit service coverage at all times in order to assure complete transfer of non-nursing functions to this section of the department. The new work schedule therefore was used for unit service personnel from the

FIGURE 2

BASIC TEN-HOUR SCHEDULE

TWO - WEEK CYCLE

	S	M	T	W	TH	F	S	S	M	T	W	TH	F	S
Employee A	-	on	on	-	-	on	on	on	-	-	on	on	-	-
Employee B	on	-	-	on	on	-	-	-	on	on	-	-	on	on

FIGURE 3

BASIC SCHEDULE OF DAYS TO BE WORKED
GROUP A — Rotating & Evening Personnel

October 1970 - January 1972

	S	M	T	W	T	F	S	S	M	T	W	T	F	S	S	M	T	W	T	F	S	S	M	T	W	T	F	S
1970																												
Oct., Nov.		19	20			23	24	25			28	29				2	3			6	7	8			11	12		
Nov., Dec.		16	17			20	21	22			25	(26)				30	1			4	5	6			9	10		
70 71																												
Dec., Jan.		14	15			18	19	20			23	24	(25)			28	29			(1)	2	3			6	7		
Jan., Feb.		11	12			15	16	17			20	21				25	26			29	30	31			3	4		
Feb., Mar.		8	9			12	13	14	(15)		17	18				22	23			26	27	28			3	4		
Mar., Apr.		8	9			12	13	14			17	18				22	23			26	27	28			31	1		
Apr., May		5	6			9	10	11			14	15				19	20			23	24	25			28	29		
May		3	4			7	8	9			12	13				17	18			21	22	23			26	27		
May, June		(31)	1			4	5	6			9	10				14	15			18	19	20			23	24		
June, July		28	29			2	3	4	(5)		7	8				12	13			16	17	18			21	22		
July, Aug.		26	27			30	31	1			4	5				(9)	10			13	14	15			18	19		
Aug., Sept.	22			25	26				30	31			3	4	5	(6)		8	9				13	14			17	18
Sept., Oct.	19			22	23				27	28			1	2	3	(·)		6	7				(11)	12			15	16
Oct., Nov.	17			20	21				25	26			29	30	31			3	4				8	9			12	13
Nov., Dec.	14			17	18				22	23		(25)	26	27	28			1	2				6	7			10	11
71 72																												
Dec., Jan.	12			15	16				20	21			24	(25)	26			29	30		(1)		3	4			7	8

Note: a. Holidays are circled.

b. Weekend of August 21 & 22 is split and weekend pattern is shifted at that point in order to equitably distribute holiday work.

c. Assignment of shifts on these days and variation from basic pattern necessitated by changes in personnel or special circumstances will be posted at 4 week intervals.

Note split weekend and subsequent shift of weekends off to accommodate holidays.

program's inception. Many unit service management programs had experienced great difficulty and delay in extending their services beyond the daytime hours, so we decided to initiate our program on the night shift. We advertised in the local newspaper for personnel to work a ten-hour shift (9 p.m. to 7 a.m.) seven nights of every two-week period.

The response was tremendous, and we had more than enough applicants to cover the night shift. When we were ready to extend the unit service program to the day shift, we again had little difficulty in obtaining personnel. In spite of some initial resistance, most of the full-time unit clerks, who were to be transferred to Unit Services at that time, agreed to work the ten-hour schedule, including every other weekend, although they had never before been required to work weekends. A few could not work the schedule, but the problem was usually one of transportation rather than of unwillingness to go on the ten-hour schedule.

Evaluation of the Results

In the beginning there was considerable resistance to the length of a ten-hour shift. After having worked the schedule for a few weeks, however, the employees discovered the advantages of the number of additional days off and became firm advocates of the system. Most employees talked freely about the advantages and thus encouraged others to try the schedule. Many employees who had worked four days a week on a part-time basis went on the new schedule full time even though it required rotation to an evening or night shift whenever needed.

The part-time personnel who worked less than eight hours per shift seemed most threatened by the changes, primarily because they felt that they might lose their jobs. Because we believed in the potential effectiveness of the new schedule for both personnel and patient care, we agreed to give preference to personnel who would work the schedule and to risk losing those who could not work it and were unwilling to move to another unit or to work on an "on-call" basis. Most part-time personnel had been regularly assigned to one unit, but this assignment would no longer be assured unless they worked the new schedule. Although we believed that part-time employees could make a valuable contribution to patient care and that we should establish schedules that would make it possible for them to work, we also felt that part-time schedules had to complement the full-time schedules because of the problems that would be created in the full-time schedules if the two were not complementary.

Some part-time nurses with long service felt that the new requirements were unfair and they appealed to physicians for support. Physicians who did not fully understand the problems or the schedule tended to amplify the complaints. In spite of this problem, however, we were able to proceed with implementation because those who had tried the schedule were so enthusiastic. Less than a year after initiation, most personnel on the inpatient units and in the emergency room were on the ten-hour schedule.

Personnel working the schedule were surveyed twice, after six months and again a year later. Only one in each of the five work groups wished to return to the old schedules. The others were quick to point out the advantages of the new schedules—primarily the extra days off and the three-day weekends along with the absence of single days off and long work stretches. A few employees mentioned occasional fatigue toward the end of a ten-hour shift, expecially the last of three in a row, but most of them indicated that fatigue was considerably less than under the old system. There were also many comments about greater involvement in activities away from the hospital, something that had not been possible before. A few even said that they felt as if they were having a vacation every week.

Perhaps the greatest problem was that of communication, with physicians as well as between the complementary employee groups. The head nurses and the unit service leaders were included in the work schedule from the beginning, but it soon became apparent that there were not enough strong leaders for the complementary groups on each unit. As a result, personnel who were not in the work group with their head nurse or unit service leader felt frustrated, a feeling which was shared by the head nurses and the unit service leaders as well. In some instances, nurses were not adequately prepared, and physicians' questions were answered with the response, "I don't know; I haven't been here for two days," rather than with a more helpful response. Consequently, some physicians and nurses felt that patient care was adversely affected. At the same time, other nurses recognized the significant improvement in staffing and subsequent reduction of problems during the late afternoon hours and on weekends. This, they felt, facilitated better overall care for patients. Several head nurses and unit service leaders altered their schedules so that they worked with both groups regularly, but these changes necessitated additional changes in schedules for the leaders in the complementary groups at the same time. Some of the problems were alleviated by these schedule changes. Although we had anticipated these problems, we had underestimated their severity. At one point, head nurses and unit service leaders were asked to return to the traditional schedule. Many of them resisted even though they had been quite vocal about the problems resulting from their use of the new system. For the most part they like the ten-hour work schedule.

The communication problems we experienced might not have existed had we had enough persons capable of providing strong leadership in each work group. In situations in which a strong leader is not available for each work group total responsibility for leadership of a unit should probably be assigned to one person, and this person's schedule should allow for interaction with both work groups.

Some nurses questioned the ability to provide continuity of patient care under this schedule. We deceive ourselves if we assume that the traditional schedule really provides for this continuity. Under the new work schedule it is possible to assign a patient to one or the other of two complementary groups of employees rather than to a succession of constantly changing groups. This arrangement should actually facilitate continuity rather than impede it.

Conclusion

A restructured work week is not a solution to all staffing problems, but it can help to resolve many of them. Neither is there one schedule that will work for all health care agencies. Any agency, or department thereof, that provides services for a period of ten or more consecutive hours per day may benefit from changing the structure of the work schedule; however, each agency must develop a plan to meet its own needs as well as the needs of present or potential employees.

Simplification of scheduling procedures and better distribution of personnel could result in a significant cost reduction. The simplicity of the schedule allows someone other than a nurse to plan and prepare work schedules. The longer shifts would increase the number of nursing care hours available on weekends and holidays by as much as 25 percent. This increase should reduce the need to supplement the regular staff on weekends and holidays, thereby reducing the cost of additional personnel or overtime. Concurrently, absenteeism and turnover may be reduced. In some hospitals the cost for staffing at adequate levels 24 hours per day, seven days per week, would be less under a restructured work week schedule than it would be under traditional scheduling practices. In most hospitals that now allow all employees alternate weekends and holidays off, such staffing would not result in greater cost.

An employee who now works 37.5 hours per week and who also receives ten paid holidays off each year is actually working 1762.5 hours per year, or an average of 36 hours in each of the 49 work weeks. If this employee is willing to work a longer shift but fewer days per year, to accept a different arrangement for holiday payment, and to participate in regularly scheduled inservice education programs at times when not assigned patient care responsibilities, the same average number of work hours per year could be maintained. For many nurses, 40 to 60 more days off each year combined with a stable, predictable schedule that alternates work periods of reasonable length with adequate rest periods would be very attractive.

Clinical Staffing With a 10-Hour Day, 4-Day Work Week

Jeannine Bauer

This article presents a new perspective in staffing schedules. It provides an attractive method of cyclical staffing whereby nurses employed in a full-time position work 10 hours a day and only 4 days a week, with every other week-end off. It presents the philosophy, objectives, and purpose of developing this concept of staffing, and measures its merits and disadvantages. The basic steps of planning, directing, and implementing this type of scheduling is outlined to meet the best possible balance between the needs of the patient and the needs of the employee.

Jeannine Bauer, at the time this article was published, was Clinical Coordinator of the Intensive Care Unit, Saint Elizabeth Community Health Center, Lincoln, Nebraska. The article is reprinted from JONA, November-December 1971.

Who would have thought that a 10-hour day, 4-day work week with every other weekend off duty would exist for nurses? But this working pattern is now a reality for nursing personnel in the Intensive Coronary Care Unit at Saint Elizabeth Community Health Center in Lincoln, Nebraska.

After experiencing problems in planning schedules which met the needs of both staff and patients, we decided to investigate the feasibility of a major change in staffing. Our objectives were equitable distribution of hours, predictable work schedules, and every other weekend off. We also hoped to reduce the time spent in making and maintaining schedules. After considerable research and study we decided to experiment with the cyclic staffing defined by Price.[1] It seemed to permit the best possible balance between the needs of patients and the needs of staff.

The concept of a 10-hour day is being discussed widely in this country. At first we thought it impractical, but considering the special staffing needs of our Intensive Coronary Care Unit, some potential benefits seemed possible. As primary consideration, the 10-hour day, 4-day week appeared to provide adequate staff coverage within an established budget. Initial work with imaginary schedules proved this was feasible.

At this point we began to involve the staff. We discussed the merits and the disadvantages with all the special care area nurses. We asked them whether working the extra 2 hours each day would disrupt their established daily or weekly routine? Would a 10-hour day with the known physical and mental stress of an intensive care area prove fatiguing? During the discussions we carefully emphasized the disadvantages to prevent the readily apparent advantages from overshadowing all else.

The shifts developed for the 10-hour day were 7:00 A.M. to 5:30 P.M., 1:00 P.M. to 11:30 P.M., and 9:00 P.M. to 7:30 A.M. The overlap was purposely planned to provide adequate coverage for employee meals and rest breaks, to provide additional coverage during the peak work periods, and to provide coverage for planned staff development projects.

To determine the cyclic schedule, we divided our staff into three classifications, *basic, complementary,* and *float.*

The basic or minimal staff consists of the smallest number of fully oriented, full-time or part-time personnel required to staff the unit. All personnel in this class rotate shifts, except for the Team Leader and for personnel employed on permanent evening or night shifts. These personnel are all assured a cyclic pattern.

The complementary staff supplements the basic staff group and provides the *flexibility* necessary to meet short-range needs or unexpected changes in the pattern, such as unexpected terminations, vacations, or holidays. Personnel in this group are not assured a cyclic pattern. This staff consists of the most recently employed personnel assigned to the unit, those who require orientation and supervised clinical experience. Personnel classified in this group are not clinically prepared to function in a charge position, but they are assigned hours whereby they will be provided the necessary supervision. They may advance to the basic staff group as a vacancy occurs and as clinical knowledge and skill have been acquired. Following is an example of the complementary staff schedule; they repeat their schedule every two weeks on a cyclical basis.

S	M	T	W	T	F	S
2	2	X	1	1	X	X
X	1	1	X	X	2	2

Code: 1 = 7:00 A.M. to 5:30 P.M.
         2 = 1:00 P.M. to 11:30 P.M.   X = Days off

The float staff provides the flexibility to meet service needs resulting from absenteeism, vacations, and holidays or from fluctuation of the patient census or the classification of patient needs. This staff consists mainly of part-time personnel who report to the central staffing office and are assigned from the "float pool." They are oriented and trained to function in the Intensive Coronary Care Unit. (Part-time personnel are required to work every other weekend.)

In our cyclical schedule all personnel are provided every other weekend off, and single days are frequently added to weekends. No employee is scheduled for more than four consecutive 10-hour shifts in a row. All have at least 14 hours free between any shift. Those who rotate within the basic staff group are given a 4-day weekend every 6 weeks.

Shift rotation is on a 6-week cycle; 2½ consecutive weeks of days, 1½ weeks of evenings, and 2 weeks of nights with at least one day off before changing from one shift to another. Shift rotation is required for all personnel, with the exception of those assigned permanent evenings or nights. At present the number of staff that prefers evenings or nights is not adequate to cover these shifts, so rotation is required.

Following is an example of the basic staff schedule designed for six nurses. Each rotates through the entire 6-week cycle and then repeats the schedule.

S	M	T	W	T	F	S
X	X	1	1	X	1	1
1	1	X	X	1	1	X
X	X	1	1	X	2	2
2	2	X	2	2	X	X
X	X	3	3	3	X	3
3	3	X	X	3	3	X

Code: 1 = 7:00 A.M. to 5:30 P.M.
        2 = 1:00 P.M. to 11:30 P.M.
        3 = 9:00 P.M. to 7:30 A.M.   X = Days off

A pilot project involving cyclic staffing was begun on a 42-bed surgical area several months previously, so that the staff had a chance to discuss merits and disadvantages with others beforehand. This second phase, utilizing the 10-hour day, began on February 12, 1971. Six months later we were able to make some definitive statements about the workability of the plan.

Personnel are impressed with cyclic staffing because they know their hours and days off months in advance by means of the posted schedule. Short work stretches are a bonus. Long weekends and extra days off are especially attractive to nurses with families and children. Overtime is practically nonexistent. The overlap of the shifts eliminates this need. Absenteeism and employee turnover has been reduced. Vacations and trips can be planned according to the rotation. Requests for particular days off have been nonexistent. Morale has improved, and we have been able to provide adequate coverage within our projected staffing budget. Personnel have additional time to schedule and attend team conferences, to develop written care plans, and to research current literature. Scheduled classes pertinent to the care of intensive and coronary care patients are now provided on-duty time for preclass reading and preparation.

The main problem predicted for the 10-hour day was fatigue, and it does occur, but not as frequently as anticipated. The stress is relieved by the overlap of the oncoming shift. A few employees comment that they become tired from longer days, but they do not wish to switch back to the 5-day week. The long weekends and extra days off appear to be more appealing than the conventional schedule.

The Nebraska Wage and Hour Law required certain policies. No one was scheduled for more than four 10-hour shifts during any 7-day week. Nonexempt employees are paid overtime for hours worked in excess of 40 in the work week. That work week begins on Sunday and ends on Saturday. We have found that using Sunday as the first day of the week is an advantage. It increases flexibility in scheduling by providing the largest number of possible hourly schedules. The weekend for all shifts is Saturday and Sunday.

The hourly equivalent of regular benefits is used in scheduling vacations, holidays, and sick leave. Holidays are not considered such a "necessity" now because the long weekends and extra days are being provided. If nonscheduled days off are necessary, the employee assumes the initiative and responsibility for securing comparable replacement by exchanging shifts with her coworkers. The arrangement must, of course, be verified and approved by her supervisor.

We plan to continue to evaluate the program. Nurses in other areas have expressed interest in this work schedule but, although cyclic scheduling will be implemented in other areas, we have no definite plans for installing the 10-hour day in those areas. In other areas we see no justification for the overlap of shifts as it exists in the special care areas because of the unique peaks of activity and the sophisticated continuing education needs experienced there.

Our experience with the 10-hour day has been successful. Staffing needs are being met, and the nurses are experiencing a measurable increase in off duty time, time for families, leisure, social activities, and for continuing education.

REFERENCE

1. PRICE, E.M. *Staffing for Patient Care.* Springer Publishing Company, New York, 1970.

Community Nursing Administration: Quantifying Nursing Utilization

by Charmaine L. Kissinger

Charmaine L. Kissinger, R.N., M.S.N., is Assistant Project Director, Community Nursing Services of Philadelphia. The article is reprinted from JONA, September-October 1973.

A study is described which was conducted in a community nursing agency to quantify nurses' activities in such a way that the administrative staff can better plan for the utilization of field nurses.

Americans are much more aware of their health rights, and those who have not previously had equal opportunity for health care are now beginning to demand it. The delivery of health care services is being scrutinized by many individuals and groups in this country. Through the passage of social legislation, ever-increasing numbers of citizens are becoming eligible for health care services. Federal and state agencies are insisting on accountability from health professionals to insure that quality service is provided. The National Advisory Commission on Health Manpower, in reviewing many of the problems that impinge on the health care system, concluded, "As effective demand exceeds the capacity of available manpower to provide services in traditional ways, and as performance standards increase, tasks and responsibilities will need redefinition" [1].

A community nursing agency in a large metropolitan city, realizing that its goals of providing nursing care, promoting health, and preventing disease are becoming increasingly complex and difficult to achieve, resolved to reassess the role of the community nurse. Administrative staff sought answers to questions such as: Given the nursing staff available, is each nurse fulfilling her role to optimum capacity? Can the nurse extend herself further? Are there tasks which she is currently doing that could be done by persons with less training? Can a way be found to quantify her activities? The pursuit of answers to these questions is the focus of the study described in this paper.

It was recognized that the agency did not have an objective way in which to determine the kind of staff it needed to meet the growing demands of the community. Staffing patterns at the agency have developed experientially rather than scientifically. A time study, done twice yearly for a two-week period, is used primarily for cost accounting. The staff nurse records, to the nearest five-minute interval, the amount of time devoted to specified activities. These activities are very broad and do not provide the detailed information needed to study utilization of the nurse's time. For example, one category is entitled "Preparation and Postactivity." Time charged to this item includes bag preparation, obtaining and reviewing records, making telephone calls, etc. Figures from a recent time study reveal that approximately 31 minutes were related to preparation and postactivity, while 23 minutes was the average time spent with each patient. These figures are interesting, but they do not give enough significant information on which to base changes in assignments.

By peer review a record audit is done four times yearly on a sample of all nursing records. The purpose of the audit is to analyze and evaluate the appropriateness of the service given to a specific patient. It does not serve as a tool by which a judgment can be made regarding the level of training a staff member needs to perform a given activity.

Both the time study and record audit serve useful purposes, but neither provides enough information for redefining tasks and responsibilities. Although these methods may have the potential for supplying information about utilization, both would have to be significantly changed if they are to be used for the purpose of task analyses. Wald and Leonard suggest that "pressure for the nurse to act—not to stop and think—is very real [2]. They contend that this constant demand for action has created practices and theories based on untested assumptions. As an alternative approach, they recommend that an analysis of clinical experiences be used to develop future concepts.

A review of the literature revealed no method whereby the activities performed by community health nurses can be documented to answer the questions posed [3–11]. It hypothesized that to fully utilize personnel and to better predict the level of personnel needed to meet future agency demands, an analysis of current tasks is a prerequisite. The first step in reaching this end is the development of a way to study the activities of the community health nurse.

STUDY METHODS AND ENVIRONMENT

The author functioned as the investigator for this applied research study. She served as a nonparticipant observer in the collection of data needed to develop a methodology. Justification for using an observer was twofold. First, subjectivity in collecting information could be kept at a minimum. Second, some practical questions could be answered regarding the effect of an outside observer in the office and home setting. Can the nurse perform in her usual manner with an observer present? Is the nurse-patient relationship influenced by the presence of an observer? Strict discipline on the observer's part had to be maintained to prevent intrusion into the situation observed.

In June 1971, the agency had a total of 54 community health nurses and 18 community health nurse trainees deployed in the nine health districts of the city. These figures do not reflect the total staff employed by the agency, but rather that group of nurses who visit in the home. The community health nurse, by agency definition, is one who has completed a bachelor's degree at an accredited college or university with major course work in nursing or nursing education, including or supplemented by an accredited training program in community health nursing. The trainee is a person who has completed a diploma program at an accredited school of nursing and is obtaining credits toward a bachelor's degree in nursing at an accredited college or university.

As an expedient measure, since the inclusion of all health districts would have entailed undue time and expense, only one district was chosen for the first phase of the study. From this district 7 community health nurses and 1 trainee participated. Approximately 156,500 persons live in this most densely populated area of the city. A total range of disease entities and related social and economic conditions are known to exist in this population. At the time of this study, the health district had been designated as a future family-care center where integrated rather than categorical services would be available to the community. Heretofore, the city's health centers provided mainly preventive services for specific health and disease categories. With the addition of diagnostic and treatment services, covering the total spectrum of health needs, the nursing agency has envisioned a greatly increased work load for their nurses. This factor added impetus to the necessity of a task analysis.

Prior to the observation period, a meeting was held with the community nursing staff (7 community health nurses and 3 trainees), their supervisor, and the district nursing supervisor. An explanation of the study and the methodology to be used was received with an unusual amount of enthusiasm. The staff nurses expressed concern about the amount of time spent in other than direct nursing activities and indicated a willingness to participate. The essential information conveyed to the staff was as follows: "Observations, for the purpose of collecting data, will take place within the next four-week period. This time is prior to most vacations, least affected by illness and weather patterns, and free of other studies. The days chosen will be Monday through Friday, when the work days are the most normal. The days will be chosen at random as will the name of the nurse to be observed that day. Thus preparation which might be made for the observer's benefit can be kept at a minimum. It is important that tasks be performed as exactly as normally. Performance is not being evaluated. No names will be recorded on the log. The observer is attempting to obtain a sample of the many tasks a nurse is called upon to do."

Observations began within a week of the meeting and extended for a four-week period. Two Mondays, Tuesdays, and Wednesdays, and one Thursday and Friday were the results of random selection of the observation days. The length of service of the nurses who participated ranged from nine months to twenty years, with a mode of two years. Observations, which began at 8:30 A.M. and ended at 5:00 P.M., were recorded on the log sheet. The log provided a sequential account, by minutes, of every activity performed during the specified time period. The observer described in narrative form what she saw the nurse doing. The diagnosis of the patient for whom the activity was being carried out was noted. A comment column provided space for any needed explanations. The nurse therefore was able to proceed with her duties without explaining her movements to the observer. If a diagnosis was needed, the information was obtained from the patient's record. Because there was travel time between each visit, the nurse used this opportunity to describe patient and family situations to the observer. The observer was introduced to the patient as a nurse who was visiting with the regular nurse that day. There was no noticeable effect on nurse-patient interchange because of the presence of a third person.

FINDINGS

After eight days of observations had been recorded by the investigator, the worksheet was prepared on which data were summarized. This form allowed for a clearer concept of the categories into which activities fall, thus providing for more specific groupings of items. The list of general categories was subdivided into specific activities such as recording visit content, recording telephone conversations. These data were then converted to a written list of definitions which was coded by number. Two experienced community health nurses transcribed the information from an activity log to a work sheet, using the coded definitions. There was agreement as to the definitions needed to

TABLE 1.

TASK ANALYSIS AND DEFINITIONS OF TERMS

1. Written communication: Activity which encompasses tasks concerned with the record keeping necessary to maintain continuity of patient care and administrative control.
   a. Daily route sheet
   b. Recording visit content
   c. Recording telephone conversations
   d. Recording information from other sources: medical records, messages, etc.
   e. Summarizing for discharge/periodic
   f. Reviewing records for planning including tickler file, orders, medical records
   g. Completion of forms: Medical assistance, financial data, source and contact sheet
   h. Writing information exchange
   i. Writing interagency communication
   j. Request for service
   k. Communicable disease history
   l. Referral to health protection representative
   m. Initial or renewal of physician's orders
   n. Home health aide plans
   o. Mechanics: Compiling records, securing medical or nursing records, filing, taking forms to clerks
   p. Other tasks:
2. Preparation for visit: Activity which includes preparing for the home visit, as well as preparatory arrangements to other agencies and clinics.
   a. Bag preparation
   b. Enteric kits, special equipment
   c. Weekend work: work sheet, records, etc.
   d. Preparation for other services: Making clinic appointments, referral to welfare agencies, etc.
   e. Review of resource information: Procedure review, textbook, etc.
   f. Other tasks:
3. Telephoning: Activity which includes the use of the telephone to or from any source when it relates to the care or welfare of the patient.
   a. Hospital: Medical/social/nurse coordinator
   b. Health/welfare organization
   c. Patient/family
   d. Private M.D.
   e. Within center
   f. Central office—Nursing
   g. Central office—Other health service departments
   h. Home health aide
   i. Other health districts, specify contact: PHN, P. T., O. T., nutritionist, etc.
   j. Agency or supplier for equipment needs
   k. Other tasks:

4. Discussion: Activity which is an informal, unplanned meeting between two or more individuals relating to patient/family care.
   a. Supervisor
   b. Home health aide
   c. Health program representative
   d. Physical therapist
   e. Occupational therapist
   f. Information and referral nurse
   g. Physician
   h. Nutritionist
   i. Staff nurse
   j. Other tasks:
5. Conference: Activity which is a planned meeting between two or more individuals relating to patient/family care.
   a. Supervisor
   b. Home health aide/supervisor
   c. Interdisciplinary team
   d. Nursing team
   e. Consultant: designate
   f. Other tasks:
6. Patient: Activity which is done directly for or with the patient/family within the home or clinic setting. The subdivisions are broad in nature and are intended to imply introduction to the family, preparation and after care of equipment, etc.
   a. Therapeutic care: Including bathing, hypodermic, dressing, other treatment
   b. Assessment of patient's physical/emotional needs
   c. Social assessment: Housing, financial, employment factors
   d. Family assessment: Physical/social/emotional needs of family members
   e. Health supervision: Teaching, guiding, counseling to increase patient/family competence
   f. Demonstration of care to family/friend
   g. Disease investigation: CD, Tbc., etc.
   h. Environmental evaluation: Safety factors, physical, equipment
   i. Home health aide supervision
   j. Other:
   k. Absent visit
7. Miscellaneous: Activity which does not directly relate to the care of the patient.
   a. Time sheet, leave request
   b. Coffee break
   c. Personal
   d. Staff association
   e. General staff meeting
   f. Public relations: Speaking to outside groups
   g. Car maintenance
   h. Other tasks:
8. Travel
   a. Self-explanatory: Charge cost center to which visit is being made

TABLE 2

TABLE 2
ESTIMATED PERCENT OF TOTAL ACTIVITIES AND TOTAL TIME BY TYPE OF ACTIVITY AND TIME IN MINUTES

Time In Minutes	Records No. %	Preparation No. %	Telephone No. %	Written Communications	Discussion No. %	Conference No. %	Patient Care No. %	Education No. %	Misc. No. %	Total[b] No. %
1-4	87 58%	12 71%	52 63%	4 44%	34 65%		8 15%		18 18%	215 46%
5-9	39 26%	5 29%	22 27%	5 56%	12 23%		4 8%		35 35%	122 26%
10-14	16 11%		6 7%		5 10%		8 15%		29 29%	64 14%
15-19	4 3%		2 2%				10 19%		3 3%	19 4%
20-24	3 2%				1 2%	1 50%	11 21%		5 5%	21 5%
25-29							6 11%		1 1%	7 2%
30-34							3 6%		1	4 1%
35-39							1 2%		2	3 1%
40-44							0			1
45-49							1 2%		1	2
50-54							1 2%			2
55-59						1 50%			1 1%	6 1%
60 and over									5 5% 2 2%	2
Number of Activities	149	17	82	9	52	2	53	0	102	466
Percent of Total Activities	32%	4%	18%	2%	11%	-1%	11%	0%	22%	100%
Estimated No. of Minutes[a]	816	65	390	45	251	79	950	0	1393	Total Time 3989
Percent of Total Time	20%	2%	10%	1%	6%	2%	24%	0%	35%	Total Percent 100%

a - Estimated Time = Median of time categories times frequencies.
b - Percent to nearest whole numbers, percent less than 1 not reported.

describe the narrative information appearing on the log. Discussion of the first draft of definitions with agency personnel led to further clarification of the terms (Table 1).

The percentages of tasks, by activity and by time, as shown on Table 2, gave an indication of any additional breakdown of items needed. For example, the category Miscellaneous accounted for 35 percent of the estimated total time. However, 55 percent of the time in this category was devoted to travel, so a separate category was established for that item. The category of Written Communications, having occurred only 1 percent of the total time, was therefore included within the Records category. Although Education did not account for any of the nurses' time, it was included since the subdivisions are activities in which the nurses usually take part. The observation period had taken place during the summer when this activity is least likely to occur.

A second draft of definitions was compiled after the above factors had been considered. To further test the accuracy and relevancy of the definitions, a trial period for use by nine assistant supervisors, one from each of the health districts, was arranged. The assistant supervisors are responsible for the supervision of nursing activities within an assigned geographic area of the health district, as well as for the implementation of the nursing programs within the area. These nine observers were chosen at random in those districts which had more than one assistant supervisor assigned to field staff. Nine community health nurses who were to be observed were randomly selected from each district as well.

The instructions given the assistant supervisors by the investigator included the following information: "The purpose of the trial period is to determine the accuracy and relevancy of the definitions and to test the practicality of coding the nurses' activities onto a worksheet. The worksheet has been designed to include identifying information such as the nurse's name, the date of the observation, and the time the observation began (Table 3). The columns on the work sheet provide space to record (1) Action—the activity in which the staff nurse is involved at a given time, by code; (2) Cost Center*—the diagnosis of the patient for whom the activity is being performed, by code; and (3) Duration—the time in minutes it takes to perform each activity. A fourth column provides space to explain any code which would otherwise be unclear.

The observation period should take place for a full work day, beginning at 8:30 A.M., and ending at 5:00 P.M."

The data collected from these observations are summarized in Table 4. Only eight of the nine worksheets are reflected, because one was not returned in time for tabulation. Several changes were brought about, following analysis of the data. The item Lunch, which was included under Miscellaneous, was deleted from the definition list. This is not a true work activity and thus somewhat distorts the information needed for a task analysis. An additional item, Clerical, was added under Discussion because of the

---

Cost Center is a term used in the Time Study to describe the patient's diagnosis. It is a term commonly used by this agency and is part of the nurse's daily record. To be consistent with agency terminology it has been retained here.

number of times it appeared as an additional description on the worksheet. The category Education was excluded because it again did not account for any time.

In discussion with the supervisors following their observation period, other suggestions were taken into account and changes were made as follows: The term Written Communications was used in place of Records and the general definition of Patient Care was expanded for further clarity. With these few exceptions, the supervisors found the definitions precise and in keeping with the work performed by the staff nurse. In comparing the results of the data collected by the observer with that collected by the supervisors, there is a consistency in both the percentage of activities and the percentage of time spent performing the various tasks.

IMPLICATIONS AND CONCLUSIONS

The purpose of this study was to design a method which would provide accurate information about the utilization of the community health nurse's time. As suggested earlier, unless detailed documentation of activities in which the nurse is engaged is obtained, planning for the future nursing needs of the community cannot be realistically accomplished. Without a comprehensive job analysis, administrative staff cannot objectively redefine the nurse's function. The assumption that a redefinition is needed is based on the knowledge that nursing needs in the community are not currently being met and that an increase in the demand for nursing care is predictable.

The methodology developed by the investigator was pretested by a group of assistant supervisors. They found the definitions reliable and valid and the worksheet practical for use in the work setting. An analysis of the results of the data illustrates that activities performed by the staff nurse and the time spent in doing these activities are measurable. Thus administration can be provided with explicit information, in quantitative terms, which will allow for objective decision making. If a task analysis of this kind were to be done on a sample of nurses in each district served by the agency, a definitive work pattern should evolve and make planning for both communities and staff more appropriate. While social, cultural, and economic factors, as well as the health indices of each community, have been used as indicators for planning, there are internal factors which also must be taken into account. These factors, it is believed, are specifically related to the means by which the agency may or may not reach its stated goals. Approximately one-third of the nurse's time is used directly with the patient. The remaining two-thirds is spent in planning and in paper work. The primary objective of the agency is the provision of direct nursing care to the community, yet the majority of the nurse's time is spent in other than direct service.

If it is shown, for example, that three-quarters of the total telephone time is wasted because the line is busy or the person being contacted is not available, is this not an indication that more appropriate personnel is needed? Similarly, an analysis of written communications demonstrates that a substantial percentage of the time is devoted to repetitive clerical tasks. However, there are indirect patient activities that must remain within the province of the nurse. She alone possesses the judgment and discrimination to carry out these activities. The task analysis method has the potential for separating specific activities within general categories and in so doing, for depicting those areas that could be delegated to lesser trained personnel. The supposition that delegation of tasks will increase the amount of nursing time for direct patient care can be determined only by future research. The additional costs for such delegation may mean more expensive but higher quality nursing care to more patients.

The addition of the patient's diagnosis to the task analysis can also aid in planning. A superficial investigation of the data from this study revealed that certain diagnoses, especially communicable diseases, required a dis-

TABLE 3. PRELIMINARY TASK ANALYSIS

Name			Month	Day	Year	Start Time	
						Hour	Minute
Action	Cost Center	Duration	Comment	Action	Cost Center	Duration	Comment

TABLE 4.
ESTIMATED PERCENT OF TOTAL ACTIVITIES AND TOTAL TIME BY TYPE OF ACTIVITY AND TIME IN MINUTES

Time In Minutes	Records No. %	Preparation No. %	Telephone No. %	Discussion No. %	Conference No. %	Patient Care No. %	Education No. %	Misc. No. %	Travel No. %	Total [b] No. %
1-4	170 75%	17 74%	54 77%	61 88%		9 12%		21 40%	12 21%	344 60%
5-9	43 19%	5 22%	11 16%	4 6%	2	15 21%		14 27%	12 21%	106 18%
10-14	14 6%		5 7%	1 1%	1	11 15%		7 13%	12 21%	51 9%
15-19	1	1 4%				9 12%		1 2%	12 21%	24 4%
20-24				1 1%		10 14%		0	3 6%	14 2%
25-29				2 3%		8 11%		0	2 4%	12 2%
30-34						5 7%		0	3 6%	8 1%
35-39						2 3%		0		
40-44						2		1		
45-49						1 1%		0		
50-54						0		1		
55-59						1		1		
60 and over								6 12%		6 1%
Number of Activities	228	22	70	69	3	73	0	52	56	573
Percent of Total Activities	40%	4%	12%	12%	1%	13%	%	9%	10%	100%
Estimated No. of Minutes[a]	911	94.5	272	268.5	26	1270.5	0	464.5	678	Total Time 3985
Percent of Total Time	23%	2%	7%	7%	1%	32%	0%	12%	17%	Total Percent 100%

a - Estimated Time = Median of time categories times frequencies.
b - Percent to nearest whole numbers, percent less than 1 not reported.

proportionate amount of office time. Control mechanisms are essential for the prevention and containment of contagious diseases, but one must ask whether a professional nurse need be involved in many of the mechanics currently in use.

The observer approach in collecting data has implications for supervisory staff as well. Although several supervisors noted that the full day of observation was time-consuming, the majority felt that they had gained meaningful insight into the abilities and needs of their staff nurses. Using this information as baseline data, the supervisor can better measure the progress an individual nurse is making. Moreover, she has some indication if the supervisory methods she is employing are effective.

If this task analysis method is used more widely, additional implications and limitations will become apparent. Future research should be directed toward the development of more exact definitions for the direct patient activities. With more specificity in these definitions, explicit standards of nursing care should be set by administrators, as a basis of comparison by which actual practice can be measured. This study is a beginning in the search for measures of efficiency and effectiveness that will enable a redefinition of the tasks and responsibilities of community health nurses.

REFERENCES

1. National Advisory Commission on Health Manpower. *Report Volume II.* Washington, D. C.: Gov. Ptg. Office, November 1967.
2. Wald, F. and Leonard, R. Towards development of nursing practice theory. *Nurs Res.,* 13 (4): 309–313, 1964.
3. Benjamin, R. A. Analysis of health care delivery by the frontier nursing service. (Unpublished paper, October 1969.)
4. Yankauer, A.; Connelly, J., Feldman, J. A survey of allied health worker utilization in pediatric practice in Massachusetts and in the United States. *Pediatrics,* 42 (5): 733–742, 1968.
5. Guidelines on short-term continuing education programs for pediatric nurse associates. *Am. J. Nurs.,* 71(3): 509–519, 1971.
6. Farrisey, R., Clinical nursing in transition. *Am. J. Nurs.,* 67 (2): 305–309, 1967.
7. Urey, B. A method for analysis of nursing tasks. *Dissertation Abst. Int.,* 30 (3): 1215B, 1969.
8. U. S. Department of Health, Education, and Welfare. *How to Study the Nursing Service of an Outpatient Department,* by Apollonia O. Adams. Public Health Service Publication No. 497. Washington, D. C.: Gov. Ptg. Office, 1964.
9. U. S. Department of Health, Education, and Welfare. *How to Study Nursing Activities In A Patient Unit.* Public Health Service Publication No. 370. Washington, D. C.: Gov. Ptg. Office, 1964.
10. Parrish, H., Bishop, F., Baker, M., Sherwood, A. Time study of general practitioner's office hours. *Arch. Env. Health* 14 : 892–898, 1967.
11. Dumas, N. S. and Muthard, J. E. Job analysis method for health-related professions: A pilot study of physical therapists. *J. Appl. Psychol.* 55 (5): 458–465, 1971.

Satisfaction of Job Factors For Registered Nurses

by Douglas A. Benton and Harold C. White

Douglas A. Benton, Ph.D. is Associate Professor and Research Coordinator of Management at Colorado State University. **Harold C. White,** Ph.D. is Professor of Management, Arizona State University, Tempe. The article is reprinted from JONA, November-December 1972.

A study of 565 registered nurses was conducted to obtain their reactions to 16 job factors. The nurses indicated that factors of greatest importance to them were safety and security, followed by social, esteem, and self-actualization factors. Pay and personnel policies were of least importance. A more useful measure was applied to the job factors by identifying how the nurses perceived these factors as being deficient, that is, how dissatisfied they were with the factors.

Nursing supervision seeks means of obtaining maximum performance from the nurses. Perhaps the most useful approach is through the identification of the needs of nurses. Once these needs are identified, supervisors can take steps to fulfill them. It is through need satisfaction that effective work performance is obtained. The consequences of not recognizing these needs can be undesirable for the patients and the hospital, as well as for the nurses. One observer has described nurses as ". . . deprived of esteem and acceptance . . . and become paralyzed. They fail to develop their potentials, conform to existing patterns and levels of performance, or detach themselves from nursing service altogether. [These failures] must have a cause not yet identified . . . ."[1]

It is the purpose here to attempt to identify these causes, at least in part, and more importantly, to suggest approaches to overcome them.

MOTIVATION OF EMPLOYEES

There is a theoretical and empirical body of knowledge to aid in the understanding of motivation and individual needs. Motivation has been defined as "the process (a) of arousing or initiating behavior, (b) of sustaining an activity in progress, and (c) of channeling activity into a given course."[2] Needs are the various physiological, sociological, and psychological requirements which are to be fulfilled for the comfort and well being of the individual.

Maslow has suggested that needs are arranged in a hierarchy. A lower level need must be satisfied, or partially satisfied, before a higher level need may emerge as a motivator. Listed in ascending order, the need categories are: (1) physiological, (2) safety and security, (3) belongingness and love, (4) esteem, and (5) self-actualization.[3] Although the hierarchical concept of needs has not been well supported in research literature, the classifications of needs are generally agreed upon.[4]

Incentives or goals are means to bring about fulfillment of needs. Incentives are the external factors that the individual perceives as possible satisfiers of his needs. As a consequence, each individual's behavior will be influenced by his personal expectation that a given incentive will fulfill a need. Therefore, the behavior we observe in others is caused by a striving for the satisfaction of needs.

Anxiety, conflict, frustration, and feelings of failure can develop within an employee when his needs are not consistent with the opportunities and requirements presented by the employing organization.

Numerous studies in the literature concern job satisfaction and morale. Zaleznik and his associates have reported elements that are repeatedly found from such surveys which influence individual satisfaction and productivity:

1. The technical organization of the group
2. The social structure of the group
3. The individual task motivation, i.e., the willingness to work hard that each member brings to and maintains toward his job
4. The rewards he receives from doing the job
5. The satisfaction he obtains from being an accepted member of the group[5]

These elements suggest the complexity of understanding and influencing morale in the work place. Further, such factors as employee age, education, and occupation can each influence expectations and job satisfaction.

Herzberg has categorized specific job aspects into major job factors. Reporting on various studies totaling several thousand employees in nonhospital occupations, these job factors, in order of importance to the employees, are:

1. Security
2. Opportunity for advancement
3. Company and management
4. Wages
5. Intrinsic aspects of job
6. Supervision
7. Social aspects of job
8. Communication

9. Working conditions
10. Benefits[6]

MOTIVATION OF NURSES

Nearly twenty years ago, Bullock concluded that both social and organizational factors are significantly related to job satisfaction and work efficiency of nurses[7]; but empirical research of nurses' job satisfactions is relatively recent. Frequently, the research reported includes the personal opinions of the authors and has limited substantive value.

Marlow, in a useful study interpreting responses from over 200 nurses in Pennsylvania, obtained the following rank order of factors important to nurses:

1. Good working conditions
2. Work that keeps you interested
3. Job security
4. Good wages
5. Full appreciation of work done
6. Tactful discipline
7. Personal loyalty to workers
8. Promotion and growth in the hospitals
9. Feeling "in" on things
10. Sympathetic help on personal problems[8]

As noted, motivation and need satisfaction may be influenced by occupation. Even within the single profession of nursing such varied influences exist. Research has indicated significant differences concerning needs and job satisfaction between medical and surgical nurses. Medical nurses preferred individual, talkative patients who needed TLC (tender, loving care), whereas surgical nurses preferred middle-aged, self-reliant patients with good prognoses.[9] Differences in personality structure between psychiatric and nonpsychiatric nurses in Veterans Administration hospitals have been identified. Psychiatric nurses tended to be more aggressive, introspective, and dominant; nonpsychiatric nurses were more ordered, deferent, and abased, tending toward a work orientation rather than a patient orientation.[10]

Compared to practical nurses, nurses aides, medical technologists, x-ray technicians, office workers, and unskilled employees, it has been found that the registered nurse:

1. Demands more of her environment
2. Wants others to give her recognition for her work in addition to receiving an internal reward for having upheld the tradition of nursing
3. Wants to be looked upon as a professional person rather than an ancillary hand to be manipulated by head nurses and physicians
4. Wants more independence in molding of and participating in her career[11]

It was concluded that nurses "want the most from their job and get the least from it and end up with the lowest average job satisfaction score."

THE STUDY

Following is a report on a survey of registered nurses to determine their responses concerning the importance and level of satisfaction of certain job factors. Sixteen job factors were categorized by a panel of 22 nurses into Maslow's need hierarchy. The physiological need category is not included. Five job factors, considered by the panel of nurses as being important but difficult to classify, are included in a separate category as Nonspecific.

The population for the study consisted of practicing registered nurses in nonfederal, general care hospitals in the metropolitan area of a southwestern city. Nurses participating were drawn from hospitals selected randomly to represent small, medium, and large institutions. Of 796 questionnaires distributed to a total population of approximately 2,000 nurses, there were 565 (71 percent) returned and usable.

Classification of the respondents by occupational group and number of respondents in each was:

Obstetrical (89)
Pediatrics (58)
Medical only (77)
Surgical (postoperative) only (85)
Medical-surgical combination (71)
Intensive care (80)
Specialties—operating, emergency, recovery room, etc. (76)
Administrative—directors, assistants, in-service, etc. (29)

A technique developed by Porter was utilized to determine the degree of satisfaction with and the importance of each job factor felt by the respondents. For each job factor the following questions were asked:

1. *How much* of the characteristic *is there now* connected with your nursing position?
2. *How much* of the characteristic do you think *should be* connected with your nursing position?
3. *How important* is this characteristic to you?

Respondents answered each question by circling a number on a rating scale from 1, indicating low or minimum amounts, through 7, indicating high or maximum amounts of the characteristic.

Responses to the questionnaire are presented in the following discussion in terms of importance: — "How important is this to me?" and deficiency (satisfaction-dissatisfaction), the difference between responses: "How much should there be?" and "How much is there now?"

IMPORTANCE OF JOB FACTORS

Table 1 presents the importance of each job factor as reported by occupational groups of nurses. The column for Rank indicates the relative importance of the factors: 1 indicates highest importance through 16 for lowest importance. Each factor will be considered in order of appearance in the table.

TABLE 1

RANKING OF JOB FACTOR IMPORTANCE BY OCCUPATIONAL GROUPS OF NURSES

Job Factor	Occupational Group								
	OB Rank	Peds. Rank	Med. Rank	Surg. Rank	M-S Rank	Int. Care Rank	Spec. Rank	Admin. Rank	Overall Rank of Importance
SAFETY AND SECURITY:									
Job security	2	3	4	6	5	6	4	4	4
Appropriateness of hours worked	10	10	6	5	10	8	10	12	9
Adequate personnel per shift	4	5	2	2	3	2	3	2	2
Physical working conditions	5	8	5	8	9	5	5	11	6
SOCIAL:									
Congenial work associates	3	2	3	3	1	4	1	6	3
Appreciation by patients	11	14	12	13	8	12	14	14	13
ESTEEM:									
Authority and responsibility to do job	6	6	8	4	4	3	6	3	5
Management recognition of nurses' personnel unit	13	11	13	12	7	13	13	7	12
SELF-ACTUALIZATION:									
Patient care	1	1	1	1	2	1	2	15	1
Promotion opportunities	16	16	16	16	16	14	16	16	16
Inservice training programs	12	12	11	10	6	7	9	4	10
NONSPECIFIC:									
Basic salary	7	4	7	6	13	9	8	9	7
Pay differential for education	14	15	15	15	15	15	15	13	15
Pay differential for experience	9	7	10	9	12	11	11	8	11
Written job descriptions	15	13	14	14	14	16	12	10	14
Written personnel policies	8	9	9	11	11	10	7	1	8

Safety and Security

Job security was ranked fourth in importance overall by all the nurses, from second in importance by obstetrical nurses to sixth in importance by surgical and intensive care nurses. Of all job factors in this category, *appropriateness of hours worked* was of least importance (9), but both surgical and medical nurses rated it relatively high (5 and 6 respectively). *Adequate personnel per shift* was ranked second of the sixteen factors, indicating the high importance given this by most nursing groups. The nursing units ranked *physical working conditions* from fifth to ninth in importance; administrative nurses ranked working conditions relatively low (11), suggesting a potential conflict in priorities between nurses in administration and the nursing units they supervise.

Social

All nursing units considered *congenial work associates* to be of relatively high importance (1 through 4); administrative nurses showed relatively less concern for this factor (6). Medical-surgical nurses gave evidence of greater concern for patient relationships, ranking *appreciation by patients* much higher (8) than did the other groups (11 through 14). For all nursing groups, relationships with fellow employees were of greater importance than were relations with patients.

Esteem

All groups ranked *authority and responsibility to do the job* in the top half of all factors listed, but there was a considerable difference in responses between that of intensive care and administrative nurses (both 3) to medical nurses (8). The nurses indicated relatively less importance for *management recognition,* but, again, there was a marked difference in the responses between the groups, ranging from medical-surgical and administrative nurses (both 7) to obstetrical, medical, and intensive care (each 13).

Self-Actualization

It is encouraging to note that *patient care* was ranked first or second in importance for all groups of practicing nurses. In contrast, administrative nurses listed patient care as fifteenth in importance of the sixteen factors. Such a difference in ranking may suggest a further potential conflict in orientation between nurses in administrative positions and the registered nurses they supervise. *Opportunities for promotion,* ranked last overall, appears to hold little importance for any of the nursing groups, even those in administration who have accepted promotions. *Inservice training programs* were regarded relatively low in order of importance for most nursing groups. Perhaps understandably, administrative nurses were most interested in training for the nurses they supervise, ranking training fourth; of the nursing units, medical-surgical (6) and inten-

sive care (7) evidenced the greatest interest. Giving least importance to training are the nurses in obstetrics and pediatrics (both 12).

Nonspecific

For nurses as a whole, *basic salary* does not occur until the seventh factor in order of importance, although salary varies considerably in importance between groups from pediatric nurses (4) to medical-surgical nurses (13). *Pay differential for education* was relatively unimportant for all nursing groups, and ranked no higher than thirteenth. Although remaining low in importance, all nursing groups were more concerned about *pay differential for experience.* As for basic salary, pediatric nurses ranked this higher than other groups (7) and medical-surgical nurses ranked it lower than the other groups (12).

Written job descriptions held little importance for the nursing units (12 through 16). Administrative nurses ranked job descriptions higher (10) than did the nursing units. Such an administrative orientation for administrative nurses continues to be indicated most dramatically in that they list *written personnel policies* as first in importance of all factors; nurses in the various units rank personnel policies from a high of 7 for nursing specialists to a low of 11 for surgical and medical-surgical nurses.

SUMMARY OF JOB FACTOR IMPORTANCE

When job factors are classified according to the need hierarchy postulated by Maslow (excluding the physiological factors), the highest average ratings for *importance,* as determined in this study, were for those factors under the Safety and Security category, which include adequate personnel per shift, job security, physical working conditions, and appropriateness of hours worked per shift. Social needs are second in overall importance, including congenial work associates and appreciation by patients. Esteem is third, for authority and responsibility to do the job and management recognition of nurses' personnel unit. Fourth is self-actualization concerning patient care, promotion opportunities, and inservice training programs. It is of interest to note that the categories were selected in importance in the same order as Maslow has listed the need categories; the lower the need category, the higher the importance given to it by the nurses. The nonspecific factors of basis salary, pay differential for education, pay differential for experience, written job descriptions, and written personnel policies are of lesser average importance than for the four need categories.

While the data are not presented in Table I, administrative nurses perceived the job factors overall to be more important than did the nurses in the units. Administrative nurses were followed in order of expressions of importance of the job factors by medical, intensive care, obstetrical, specialties, surgical, and pediatrics nurses, with medical-

TABLE 2

RANKING OF JOB FACTOR DEFICIENCIES BY OCCUPATIONAL GROUPS OF NURSES

Job Factor	Occupational Group								
	OB Rank	Peds. Rank	Med. Rank	Sug. Rank	M-S Rank	Int. Care Rank	Spec. Rank	Admin. Rank	Overall Rank of Deficiency
SAFETY AND SECURITY:									
Job security	7	9	12	11	7	11	11	11	10
Appropriateness of hours worked	16	16	15	15	14	15	15	15	15
Adequate personnel per shift	2	4	3	2	1	2	3	5	2
Physical working conditions	11	5	8	9	8	7	8	6	8
SOCIAL:									
Congenial work associates	9	10	14	14	15	12	13	16	13
Appreciation by patients	15	15	16	16	16	16	16	13	16
ESTEEM:									
Authority and responsibility to do job	14	14	13	13	13	14	14	13	14
Management recognition of nurses' personnel unit	4	7	7	7	9	8	6	8	6
SELF-ACTUALIZATION:									
Patient care	12	13	10	10	12	13	12	11	12
Promotion opportunities	3	3	6	3	5	4	4	10	4
Inservice training programs	5	1	2	4	2	3	2	2	3
NONSPECIFIC:									
Basic salary	8	8	9	6	4	5	9	9	9
Pay differential for education	5	6	5	5	9	6	7	1	5
Pay differential for experience	1	2	1	1	3	1	1	3	1
Written job descriptions	10	12	4	8	6	9	5	7	7
Written personnel policies	13	10	11	12	11	10	10	3	11

surgical giving least weight to the importance of the factors. Although the perceived differences in importance do exist, the various nursing groups tend to be more alike than different in their perceptions. There are only three job factors for which statistically significant differences occur between groups. These are patient care, adequate personnel per shift, and written personnel policies. As has been noted, the differences that do occur tend to be between administrative nurses and the other nursing occupational groups rather than between the various nursing groups themselves.

DEFICIENCIES OF JOB FACTORS

Deficiencies of job factors is of considerable practical value to those involved with the supervision of nursing units. The greater the expression of deficiency in a job factor, the greater is the implied dissatisfaction of the nurses concerning that factor and the lower the morale. Individuals with high satisfaction tend to invest more energy in their jobs than do those with low job satisfaction.

Results of expressions of deficiencies are listed in table II. Relative deficiencies for each job factor are given under the rank column, indicating the factor of greatest deficiency as 1 through the factor of least deficiency as 16.

Safety and Security

There was a mixed reaction by the nurses in their perceptions of *job security*. For most nursing groups the ranking fell between 9 and 11, indicating it was low in deficiency, that is, generally well satisfied, but both obstetric and medical-surgical nurses ranked it in the top half of the job factors listed (both 7). Hospital management appears to do an acceptable job in shift assignment as indicated to responses for *appropriateness of hours worked,* with no group rating it higher than fourteenth in deficiency. The nurses apparently recognized the need to cover all shifts and perceived the administration as being equitable in making such assignments.

On the other hand, *adequate personnel per shift,* listed second in importance (Table 1), was also second in terms of deficiency. This response would appear to indicate a priority item for the hospitals involved. It may be that this factor would not receive the attention desired by the nurses as a whole because administrative nurses did not perceive the deficiency to the same degree as did the nursing groups, ranking it fifth. The concern for adequate personnel has been found in other studies as well. It has been reported that workloads influenced the degree of job satisfaction in a major eastern city for public health nurses.[13] Another report indicated that in one hospital understaffing was a major factor leading to turnover of nurses.[14]

There is evidence that the felt deficiency may be even greater for nonmetropolitan nurses. It has been concluded in one study that general duty nurses in smaller communities are faced with greater challenge in their work because there is a greater relative scarcity of nurses, causing the nurses to increase their range of duties, and, thus, increase the chances for error.[15]

There was a marked difference in the responses by nursing groups concerning *physical working conditions,* from a ranking of 5 for pediatric nurses to a low of 8 for obstetric nurses. Such difference emphasize that the nature of duties may well influence responses concerning various factors of the job.

Social

Congenial work associates is thirteenth overall in order of deficiency. This is encouraging considering the high level of importance (3) indicated for this factor in Table 1. The greatest deficiency was expressed by obstetric (9) and pediatric (10) nurses, the least by administrative and medical nurses (both 16). An explanation for this may be that obstetrical and pediatric nurses are more likely to work individually, whereas nurses in other units are more likely to work in teams. That is, it can be expected that all nurses have a need for social interaction; some duty assignments, more than others, provide a means to satisfy that need. The importance of work group relationships for job satisfaction has been well established for numerous occupational groups.[16]

Appreciation by patients was considered as being lowest in overall deficiency. Argyris found nurses in a cancer hospital to have certain "predispositions" that might indicate they are more interested in serving others than in being rewarded for their service.[17] Such a conclusion is speculative, but it is consistent with the responses of the nurses in this study who appeared to expect little appreciation from patients and were generally satisfied with the amount they do receive.

Esteem

From an administrative standpoint, while nurses overall rated *authority and responsibility to do the job* high in importance, the amount of authority and responsibility they do have is generally considered adequate (13 or 14 for each group). The hospitals surveyed for this study may be more effective in delegation than is true of other hospitals. In the study by Marlow reported earlier, the average nurse was perceived to be in a "regulation-ridden position" requiring obedience and uncomplaining acceptance of orders and criticism. The nurses perceived their occupation as a whole to be intellectually narrowing, dominated by males, and not providing any "stepping stones" to other careers.[18]

Management recognition, listed twelfth in importance, is sixth in order of deficiency. Those expressing the greatest relative deficiency were obstetric nurses (4); the least felt deficiency was indicated by medical-surgical nurses (9). Nurses in units expressing the greatest relative dissatisfaction are indicating that those in authority—both hospital administrators and physicians—are not providing the nurses with adequate expressions of appreciation for their efforts and accomplishments.

Self-Actualization

While the factor of greatest importance to nurses overall was *patient care,* it is encouraging to note it was only twelfth overall in deficiency, indicating nurses perceive patients as being relatively well cared for. Pediatric and intensive care nurses (13) expressed the greatest satisfaction with patient care, while the greatest deficiencies were expressed by medical and surgical nurses (10).

Promotion opportunities were rated by nurses as a group as being least in importance in all factors, but was one of the most deficient (4). The greatest deficiency was indicated by obstetrical, pediatric, and surgical nurses (all ranked it 3); of the nonadministrative nursing groups, medical nurses expressed the least deficiency (6). Responses by administrative nurses indicated much less deficiency for promotion opportunities (10); this is perhaps not surprising in that they have received promotions and, therefore, were more likely to have had the opportunity to experience need satisfaction. A low ranking in importance for promotion opportunities might be explained by the low regard held for administration by nurses in some hospitals.[18] This does not explain the dissatisfaction of the nurses in this study concerning promotion opportunities. Argyris, while concluding that supervisory and head nurses did not like to direct, penalize, or check on their subordinate nurses, also found these same nurses were "upward mobile," indicating a desire for promotion.[19] In a more recent study, Gross and Brown concluded that the registered nurse is assertive and selfassured, whose personal needs and values favor the role of supervisor and overseer.[20]

Another highly deficient factor is the *inservice training program* (3 overall). The greatest felt deficiency was expressed by pediatric nurses (1), followed by medical, medical-surgical, and administrative nurses; the least felt deficiency was indicated by obstetric nurses (5). To the observer, such a strong expression of relative dissatisfaction with training might be surprising. The nurse comes into the hospital with considerable professional training; the hospital field, more than most industries, conducts a variety of training programs through the individual hospitals and the various hospital related associations. The nurses' expressions of inadequacy about these programs may be the result of their awareness of the rapid changes in their field, a concern that the topics covered in training are not appropriate to their needs, or that the training techniques used are not effective.

Nonspecific

Although *basic salary* was not considered to be of special deficiency for most nurses (9 overall), medical-surgical (4), intensive care (5), and surgical (6), express rather high concern. *Pay differential for education* was reported by the nurses to be more deficient than the basic pay received (5 overall). Greatest dissatisfaction is expressed by nurses in obstetrical, medical, and surgical units. It may not be surprising that administrative nurses (1) considered pay differential to be more deficient than do nurses in the various units because they are likely as a group to have the highest level of education. Greatest overall dissatisfaction of the sixteen job factors listed occurred for *pay differential for experience.* Nurses did not consider adequate attention was given for time in the profession of nursing, and they were indicating that this factor is the greatest source of dissatisfaction of the sixteen job factors considered. The nurses appear to be indicating that their employing hospitals have not given fair or equitable consideration to the calculation of their salary. In the study of public health nurses reported previously, it was found that pay was directly related to job satisfaction.[13] It is possible that nurses' salaries may be equitably determined, but the basis is not clearly communicated to them. Dauw concluded that while salary was not one of the most important job factors to nurses, the level of satisfaction concerning salary was enhanced by clear communication from the hospital administration.[22]

Written job descriptions, one of the factors of least importance to the nurses (14), was seventh in overall deficiency. This factor shows the least agreement between the nursing groups, ranging from fourth in deficiency for medical nurses to twelfth for pediatric nurses. It appears that duties expected of nurses are not understood, perhaps, are not communicated, equally to all nursing groups by hospital management. Administrative nurses perceived a greater deficiency in *written personnel policies* (3) than did those in the nursing units; no other group ranked it higher than tenth. The nurses in these groups may be indicating that the policies are generally clear to them, whereas the administrative nurses would prefer more complete and clear guidance to aid them in their managerial duties. The importance of policies and job descriptions has been noted elsewhere. Turnover, as evidence of dissatisfaction, has been reported to result when nurses viewed their required functions as being outside their perception of the role of nurse, thereby thwarting their needs as nurses.[23] Maryo and Lasky reported that a lack of clear definition of nursing roles and personnel policies in one hospital was of greater significance than salary in contributing to the turnover of nurses.[14]

SUMMARY OF JOB FACTOR DEFICIENCY

The group expressing the greatest feeling of overall deficiencies, therefore expressing the greatest dissatisfaction, was the pediatric nurses. In descending order of dissatisfaction were medical-surgical, specialists, medical, surgical, intensive care, and obstetrics, administrative nurses expressed the least deficiencies.

The higher the overall importance of the factors indicated by an occupational group, the less likely was the group to express a feeling of *deficiency,* and the less importance overall given to the factors, the more likely was the group to express feelings of deficiency. Of the eight occupational groups, administrative nurses indicated the greatest feeling of importance for all items, but they expressed the least feeling of deficiency; pediatric nurses were seventh and medical-surgical nurses were eighth in order of groups indicating importance of the factors, but were first and second respectively in expressions of felt deficiency.

Compared to ranking for importance, there is some change for ranking of deficiency for both individual job factors and for need categories. Safety and security, ranked first in importance, remains first in deficiency also, with adequate personnel and working conditions being of major concern to the nurses. Second in importance, but last in deficiency is expressed for social; nurses generally indicate that while congenial associates are of great importance to them, they are able to satisfy this need rather well. Esteem is third in deficiency with greatest dissatisfaction expressed concerning management recognition of nursing performance. Self-actualization, of least importance of the need categories, is second for deficiency; high dissatisfaction is indicated for opportunities for promotion and training.

The value of including the category "nonspecific" is indicated by the perception that the five job factors, taken jointly, concerning pay, job descriptions, and personnel policies, were considered the most deficient of all categories.

While certain differences in terms of deficiencies for the job factors have been noted for the various groups of nurses, only six factors show statistically significant differences: patient care, appreciation by patients, congenial work associates, inservice training programs, written personnel policies, and authority and responsibility to do the job. Again, the differences in felt deficiencies were greater between administrative nurses and the nursing groups than between the various nursing groups.

CONCLUSIONS

Generalizing from one group to another is always hazardous; however, personnel responsible for the supervision and performance of hospital registered nurses should be aware of the findings reported in this study. First, it is of high priority for each hospital to identify, for each occupational group of nurses, and for each individual nurse, those job factors considered to be of importance by the nurses. The greater the importance of a factor to the nurses, the more they will expect that factor to be adequately provided; if it is not provided, the greater will be the dissatis-

faction and the less likely is it that maximum performance will be achieved. Second, hospital management should be aware of the deficiencies felt about these factors so that corrective action can be taken. Factors of greatest deficiency and, therefore, greatest dissatisfaction, are most likely to lead to lowered performance. By the same token, individuals tend to be most motivated to overcome the areas of greatest felt deficiency if they perceive their efforts will be rewarded by the desired job factors as incentives; they will be more satisfied and will be more productive in their work.

Job satisfaction and performance of nurses can be improved by obtaining reports of their perceptions of job factor importance and deficiencies and by taking appropriate corrective action. Fortunately all, if not most, of the factors covered in this study are under the partial control of the hospital management.

REFERENCES

1. Reinkemeyer, Sister M. H. A Nursing Paradox. *Nursing Research* 17:4, 1968.
2. Young, P. T. In Phillip L. Harriman (Ed.), *The Encyclopedia of Psychology.* New York: Philosophical Library, 1946, pp. 384–385.
3. Maslow, A. H. *Motivation and Personality.* New York: Harper and Brothers, 1954, pp. 80–92.
4. Hall, D. T., and Nougaim, K. E. An Examination of Maslow's Need Hierarchy in an Organizational Setting, *Organizational Behavior and Human Performance.* 3:12, 1968.
5. Zaleznik, A., Christensen, C. R., and Roethlisberger, F. J. *The Motivation, Productivity and Satisfaction of Workers: A Predictive Study.* Division of Research, Graduate School of Business Administration. Boston: Harvard University, 1958, pp. 256–258.
6. Herzberg, F., Mausner, B., Peterson, R. O., and Capwell, D. F. *Job Attitudes: Review of Research and Opinion.* Pittsburgh: Psychological Service of Pittsburgh, 1957, p. 44.
7. Bullock, R. P. Position, Function and Job Satisfaction of Nurses in the Social System of a Modern Hospital, *Nursing Research* 2:4, 1953.
8. Marlow, H. L. The Registered Nurse and Employee Needs, *Nursing Outlook* 14:62, 1966.
9. Lentz, E. M. and Michaele, R. G. Comparisons Between Medical and Surgical Nurses, *Nursing Research* 1959.
10. Narvon, L., and Stauffacher, J. C. A Comparative Analysis of the Personality Structure of Psychiatric and Non-psychiatric Nurses. *Nursing Research* 7:64, 1958.
11. Palola, E. G., and Larson, W. R. Some Dimensions of Job Satisfaction Among Hospital Personnel, *Sociology and Social Research* 49:201, 1965.
12. Porter, L. W. A Study of Perceived Need Satisfaction in Bottom and Middle Management Jobs. *Journal of Applied Psychology* 45:1, 1961.
13. Picken, E. M., and Tayback, M. A Job Satisfaction Survey. *Nursing Outlook* 5:157, 1959.
14. Maryo, J. S., and Lasky, J. J. A Work Satisfaction Survey Among Nurses. *American Journal of Nursing* 59:501, 1959.
15. Habenstein, R. W., and Christ, E. A. *Professionalizer, Traditionalizer and Utilizer.* Columbia, Missouri: University of Missouri Press, 1955.
16. Fournet, G. P., Distefano, M. K., and Pryer, M. W. Job Satisfaction Issues and Problems, *Personnel Psychology* 19:165–183 (Summer), 1966; Estes, J. E. An Analysis of Employees' Attitudes Toward Their Working Environment. *Personnel Psychology* 16:55–67 (Spring), 1963.

17. Argyris, C. *Diagnosing Human Relations in Organizations: A Case Study of a Hospital.* New Haven, Connecticut: Yale University Labor and Management Center, 1956.
18. Georgopoulos, B., and Mann, F. C. *The Community General Hospital.* New York: Macmillan, 1962.
19. Argyris, C. *Diagnosing Human Relations in Organizations* . . .
20. Gross, P. A., and Brown, R. A. Contrasting Job Satisfaction Elements Shown for R. N.'s and L.P.N.'s, *Hospitals* 41:73, 1967.
21. Dauw, D. C. Human Factors Outrank Salary as Turnover Cause in this Hospital, *Hospital Topics* 44:65, 1966.
22. Bowden, E. A. F. Nurses Attitudes Toward Hospital Nursing Service: Implications for Job Satisfaction and Transfers Between Service, *Nursing Research* 16:246, 1967.

job satisfaction and float assignments

by barbara thomas

A pilot survey conducted to determine the job satisfaction of a selected group of professional nurses employed on a float basis revealed that 76 percent of the nurses surveyed were satisfied with floating and 24 percent were dissatisfied. The nurses were asked to delineate advantages and disadvantages of the float assignment and to suggest measures that would improve the job satisfaction of the float nurse.

Barbara A. Thomas, R.N., M.S., is on the faculty of Presbyterian Medical Center School of Nursing, Denver. The article is reprinted from JONA, September-October 1972.

As greater numbers of nurses are assigned "float duties" and are absorbed into the staffing patterns of patient care agencies, investigation of factors contributing to or detracting from job satisfaction becomes of particular interest to directors of nursing service in their evaluation of the effectiveness of the float nurse position.

The *float nurse* is defined as a registered nurse who reports to a central area at the beginning of a working shift to be assigned to different clinical units on a daily basis, depending on patient needs and staff absences. The factors inherent in this type of occupational structure have a significant influence on the job satisfaction of the float nurse. Some of these factors are related to frequent change of assignment and may be described as follows:

1. Having no single work group with which to identify leaves the float nurse on the periphery of several groups. Esther Lucile Brown stresses the importance of belonging to a small work group, since the group contributes to individual security and support and provides opportunity for social contacts.[1] Small group development is recognized as being a significant factor in general employee satisfaction.

2. Frequent change of assignment may also have an effect on the quality of nursing care. Much time may be spent in reorientation to the unit, patients, and staff and in carrying out routine responsibilities, with little time left for establishing helpful relationships with patients, exploring the problems of the patients, or adequately assessing the effectiveness of nursing intervention.

3. Performance evaluation of the float nurse may be seriously affected because of frequent changes in her assignment. Because evaluation is an important means by which the employee is provided with needed information about how she is performing, difficulties in assuring fair evaluation for the float nurse may well affect her job satisfaction.

It is entirely possible, however, that frequent change in assignment is not the major factor in determining the job satisfaction of the float nurse. Being able to arrange a work schedule around family responsibilities may overshadow any disadvantages inherent in floating. Further, floating may offer the float nurse other highly important means of satisfaction, such as the feeling that she is really *needed* wherever she is assigned, or that she is capable of meeting the challenge of a different assignment and different responsibilities each day.

The pilot study described in this paper will provide baseline information as to whether or not float nurses are satisfied with their jobs and bring into focus specific factors that warrant further study. The findings provide information about the overall job satisfaction of the float nurse as determined by the advantages and disadvantages of the position perceived by the float nurse. No attempt was made to measure specific determinants of job satisfaction for float nurses, such as reasons for floating, particular duties or responsibilities, differences in scheduling or assignment to clinical areas, or orientation procedures.

The earliest study of job satisfaction in nursing, conducted by Helen Nahm in 1940, revealed that the most important factors differentiating satisfied and dissatisfied groups of nurses were general adjustment of the individual, relationships with superiors, family and social relationships, hours of work, income, and opportunities to advance and attain ambitions.[2]

Bullock studied the position, function, and job satisfaction of nurses in the social system of a modern hospital to gain clues to factors related to the job satisfaction of nurses. He found that dissatisfactions appeared to be associated chiefly with social and organizational relationships rather than with technical functional relationships.[3]

In 1957 Pickens and Tayback conducted a study of staff nurses to determine what factors within an organization contributed to job satisfaction or dissatisfaction. This study focused on certain aspects of the job and the work environment which the investigators thought probably would affect job satisfaction, namely salary, work hours and sick leave, attitudes toward supervision, attitudes toward administration, opportunity for advancement, opportunity for active participation in program planning, relationships, and area of work. The survey revealed that overall the nurses had a high degree of satisfaction in their work. Tangible factors of salary, non-nursing aspects of work, opportunities for advancement, and workloads were found to be important in increasing or decreasing job satisfaction. Also, the staff nurse's relationships with her coworkers and supervisory and administrative personnel were found to be a vital force in the job satisfaction of the nurses who participated in the survey.[4]

Maryo and Lasky conducted a work satisfaction survey among nurses in a 500-bed hospital to determine areas that could be responsible for rapid turnover and a shortage of nurses.[5] These problem areas were identified as arising from a shortage of hospital personnel, lack of mutual trust and adequate communication between management and employee, and a poorly defined work situation. Under problems related to shortage of personnel, specific mention was made of dissatisfaction with floating. The nurses believed that understaffing necessitated floating, while floating led to frustration, lower morale, and a feeling of irresponsibility. The problems of floating were considered to be the result of the float nurse not being able to identify with a work group, causing her to have a decreased sense of responsibility about coming to work and doing her full share.[5]

More recent research on job satisfaction of nurses was carried out by Simon and Olsen.[6] Their investigation involved comparing attitudes of nursing service personnel on an experimental ward with attitudes of other personnel on the same service. Changes that had been made on the experimental ward included augmenting the nursing staff, introducing team nursing, and conducting an inservice education program. The results of this survey indicated no difference between the experimental ward and the rest of the surgical service in terms of a mean index of job satisfaction; however, nurses ranked "a good chance to do interesting work" and "opportunity to do good patient care" as among the most important factors in their jobs.

The investigator was able to locate only one study that pertained to job satisfaction of part-time nurses. Smith found that the majority of professional nurses employed on a part-time basis were satisfied with the job factors involving total competency (amount of responsibility given and amount and quality of supervision received), and were primarily dissatisfied with job factors related to hospital policy, administration, and working conditions (salary, lounge facilities, and fringe benefits).[7] Other findings indicated that adequate consideration was given to part-time nurses as to their preference of assignment to the clinical area. Their needs were considered in the scheduling of hours; the job provided an adequate amount of interest; they were able to give adequate nursing care under their working conditions; adequate recognition was given for their work; and supplies, equipment, and clinical facilities were adequate.

Because the investigator was unable to find reports in the literature on studies pertaining specifically to job satisfaction of float nurses, and because more and more health agencies are including float nurses in their staffing patterns, a preliminary study was undertaken in this area.

THE STUDY

The purpose of the study was to gather data from selected nurses employed on a float basis to determine satisfaction perceived by each regarding their particular kind of employment, to determine from the data obtained which factors are of importance to their job satisfaction, and to present data which are of interest to and can be utilized by directors of nursing service to promote job satisfaction for the professional float nurse.

Methodology

Because of the widespread use of float nurses, and because of the variety of policies of each hospital regarding them, the study was limited to a preliminary survey of float nurses in two large metropolitan hospitals, one a city-supported general hospital and the other a state-supported hospital. The city-supported hospital had a 331-bed capacity and employed 23 float nurses. The state-supported general hospital had a 425-bed capacity and employed 17 float nurses.

The sample consisted of forty nurses, the total number employed on a float basis in the two hospitals chosen for the study. Full-time or part-time nurses who occasionally were given float assignments, but were permanent staff in a specific unit, were not included in the study population.

The names of the float nurses were obtained from the nursing service departments of the participating hospitals. Each person listed was sent a questionnaire and a letter of introduction explaining the purpose of the study and assuring anonymity of responses. The questionnaire consisted of four questions; one forced-alternative question asked the subject if she was satisfied with floating and required a yes or no answer. The subject was then asked to list three or four factors about floating that she believed were advantageous, and three or four factors about floating that were not advantageous. The last question asked the respondent to suggest measures that would improve the job satisfaction of the float nurse.

Since it was designed to permit a free response from the subject rather than one limited to stated alternatives, the open-end questionnaire was chosen as the primary instrument. It provided an indicator of factors prominent in the thinking of the individual about a given issue. The greatest disadvantage in using open-ended questions is that they take more time to answer than other types of questions and that strong motivation of the subject to cooperate in the study is usually required.[8]

A two-week period was allowed for completion and return of the questionnaires. A follow-up reminder was sent to nonrespondents after the two-week period had elapsed. Two additional weeks were allotted prior to collation of the data received.

Analysis and Interpretation of Data

Approximately four weeks after the initial questionnaires had been sent, twenty-nine (75 percent) of the forty float nurses had responded. Four of the twenty-nine responses were excluded since the nurses involved were no longer in a float position and preferred not to be included in the survey. Thus, the total population of the study was twenty-five.

The first step in the analysis of responses was to classify the responses as reflecting *satisfied* or *dissatisfied* float nurses. Of the twenty-five responses, this classification resulted in nineteen (76 percent) satisfied and six (24 percent) dissatisfied. The second portion of data analysis involved categorizing advantages and disadvantages of floating as perceived by these two groups of nurses. The open-end questions were considered in separate categories for satisfied and dissatisfied nurses, and content analysis was done on all items within these categories.

The advantages and disadvantages of floating were listed according to frequency of mention. The results were as follows: Category I, advantages of floating as perceived by satisfied and dissatisfied nurses, contained eight items; Category II, disadvantages of floating as perceived by satisfied and dissatisfied nurses, contained ten items, and Category III, containing seven items, consisted of suggestions from satisfied and dissatisfied nurses on how job satisfaction for float nurses might be improved.

Comparative Interpretation of Perceived Advantages of Floating Assignment

Sixteen (84 percent) of the nurses who were satisfied with floating and four (66 percent) who were dissatisfied with floating perceived the learning experiences provided by floating as a distinct advantage. Regarding this advantage, some nurses said that floating enabled them to gain experience in a variety of nursing situations and helped them to keep up with all phases of nursing.

The second item mentioned most frequently by both groups of nurses was that the variety of work in floating assignments prevented boredom, or getting into a rut, and provided stimulation and diversity of experience. Prevention of boredom, however, appeared to be much more important to satisfied nurses since 73 percent mentioned this item as compared to only 33 percent of the dissatisfied nurses. This

finding may indicate the presence of a particular characteristic of nurses who find the float position satisfying.

Three (50 percent) of the dissatisfied nurses and six (31 percent) of the satisfied nurses listed the flexibility in arranging their hours of work as an advantage of floating. Flexible scheduling of hours seemed to be more important to dissatisfied nurses than to satisfied nurses; however, it was interesting to note that the perceived decrease in involvement in personnel problems was considered an advantage by three of the dissatisfied nurses as compared to only four of the satisfied nurses. This may indicate that the dissatisfied nurses did not wish to become involved in the administrative aspects of the day-to-day functioning of the units. This did not hold true for an equal number of the satisfied nurses.

Another interesting finding was that while seven of the satisfied nurses listed the meeting of different staff and patients as an advantage of floating, this item was not even mentioned by the dissatisfied nurses. A similar pattern can be seen in the advantage listed as "promotes understanding of other people." While 10 percent of satisfied nurses listed this item as an advantage, it too was not even mentioned by the dissatisfied nurses. From these findings it could be postulated that while the satisfied nurses appear to enjoy meeting and interacting with other persons, dissatisfied nurses experienced general lack of interest in becoming involved with others.

Satisfaction in being able to adapt and be flexible did not seem to be very important to either group since only 25 percent of the satisfied and 16 percent of the dissatisfied nurses mentioned this item as an advantage of floating. The same could be said of the next item. Only 21 percent of the satisfied nurses and 16 percent of the dissatisfied nurses believed it was an advantage to be provided with general knowledge of the entire hospital. The comparison of advantages of floating as perceived by satisfied and dissatisfied nurses is reflected in Table 1.

The most frequently listed disadvantage of floating was related to orientation. Fourteen (79 percent) of the satisfied nurses and four (66 percent) of the dissatisfied nurses mentioned that orienting themselves to different units was time consuming and frustrating. Much time was spent in locating needed supplies and in becoming familiar with procedures and routines of different units. Examples of some comments in this category were "most staff nurses do not have time or are lax in giving adequate orientation to floor routine," "allows possibility of error," and "difficult to give best patient care as one is caught up with finding where things are kept." This finding coincides with the investigator's earlier suggestion that because of frequent changes in assignment, the float nurse must spend a good deal of time in orienting and reorienting herself to different units, patients, and staff.

The second most frequently mentioned disadvantage of floating pertained to the feelings of insecurity float nurses had due to a lack of familiarity with the practice area to which they were assigned. They felt less confident in dealing with emergencies and did not like to be in charge while unfamiliar with the patients, personnel, and doctors. Forty-eight percent of the satisfied nurses and thirty-three percent of the dissatisfied nurses listed factors related to insecurity as being a disadvantage of floating. From this finding it could be postulated that security in the work situation is an important

TABLE 1

Comparative Frequency and Percentage Distribution of Advantages of
Floating as Perceived by Satisfied and Dissatisfied Nurses

Item	Frequency of Mention		Percentage Distribution	
	Satisfied Nurses	Dissatisfied Nurses	Satisfied Nurses, %	Dissatisfied Nurses, %
Provides increased learning and experience in all areas of nursing	16	4	84	66
Provides variety, preventing boredom	13	2	73	33
Provides flexible scheduling of hours	6	3	31	50
Decreases involvement in personnel problems of units	4	3	21	50
Provides opportunity to meet different staff and patients	7	-	37	-
Provides satisfaction in being able to adapt and be flexible	5	1	26	16
Provides general knowledge of entire hospital	4	1	21	16
Promotes understanding of others	2	-	10	-

consideration for float nurses.

It was interesting to note that not knowing the patients was seen as a disadvantage by only 16 percent of the dissatisfied nurses as compared to 42 percent of the satisfied nurses. For the next item, however, only 26 percent of satisfied nurses saw lack of continuity of patient care as a disadvantage of floating compared to 33 percent of dissatisfied nurses. It would seem that knowing the patients would be an important factor in continuity of patient care; therefore one would expect to see the same pattern of response to this item by both groups. From the findings of this survey, it could be postulated that both satisfied and dissatisfied nurses are either ambivalent about the effect floating has on patient care or they do not see any relationship between knowing the patients and continuity of care.

None of the dissatisfied nurses mentioned that floating assignments cause difficulties in nurse-doctor relationships, as compared to seven (37 percent) of the satisfied nurses. This could indicate that satisfied nurses place greater importance on being able to establish good relationships with the doctors, whereas factor is not of concern to dissatisfied nurses.

Twenty-one percent of the satisfied nurses and thirty-three percent of the dissatisfied nurses mentioned not being able to develop a sense of belonging as a disadvantage of floating.

Although the response to this item is not significantly strong by either group, it does serve to support Esther Lucile Brown's belief that not belonging to a small work group might be a source of job dissatisfaction.[9]

The staff attitudes toward float nurses was seen as a disadvantage by a significant number of dissatisfied nurses (66 percent), while only 5 percent of the satisfied nurses mentioned it. The dissatisfied nurses indicated they disliked having to work hard and being assigned busy work or the sickest patients while the other nurses rested. They also believed they were shown a lack of understanding by other staff and were expected to perform with a perfection not expected from regular personnel. Thus, while dissatisfied nurses did not seem to desire involvement with the staff on the units to which they were assigned, they did consider the attitudes of the staff to be very important. The opposite could also be postulated, however, in that perhaps poor staff attitudes toward float nurses have resulted in the dissatisfied nurses not wanting to become involved with the personnel on the different units. This also could be said of the next item: "unfair evaluation by peers." Again, a much larger number of dissatisfied nurses (33 percent) mentioned this item as compared to 10 percent of the satisfied nurses.

Not knowing other staff members did not seem to be a

TABLE 2

Comparative Frequency and Percentage Distribution of Disadvantages
of Floating as Perceived by Satisfied and Dissatisfied Nurses

Item	Frequency of Mention		Percentage Distribution	
	Satisfied Nurses	Dissatisfied Nurses	Satisfied Nurses, %	Dissatisfied Nurses, %
Having to orient self to different units	14	4	79	66
Causes sense of insecurity in float nurse	9	2	48	33
Not knowing patients	8	1	42	16
Lack of continuity of patient care	5	2	26	33
Difficulties in nurse-doctor relationships	7	-	37	-
Cannot develop sense of belonging	4	2	21	33
Poor staff attitudes toward float nurse	1	4	5	66
Unfair evaluation by peers	2	2	10	33
Not knowing other staff	2	1	10	16
Poor utilization of float nurses	1	1	5	16

significant disadvantage since it was mentioned by only 10 percent of satisfied nurses and 16 percent of dissatisfied nurses. Only 5 percent of the satisfied nurses and 16 percent of the dissatisfied nurses listed poor utilization of float nurses as a disadvantage of floating. Comments relating to this item included "seldom permitted to work in the position for which the nurse was trained and having to function below one's qualifications."

COMPARATIVE INTERPRETATION OF PERCEIVED DISADVANTAGES OF FLOATING ASSIGNMENTS

Comparison of the disadvantage of floating as perceived by satisfied and dissatisfied nurses is reflected in Table 2.

COMPARATIVE INTERPRETATION OF SUGGESTIONS FOR IMPROVEMENT OF JOB SATISFACTION FOR FLOAT NURSES

It was interesting to note that of the total number of respondents to the questionnaires, 63 percent of the satisfied nurses and all of the dissatisfied nurses offered suggestions for improving job satisfaction for the float nurse. Table 3 reflects the comparison of these suggestions by satisfied and dissatisfied nurses.

Limiting the number of areas in which a float nurse will function seemed to be more important to dissatisfied nurses since 50 percent made this suggestion while only 15 percent of the satisfied nurses mentioned it. Fairly even percentages of both groups considered a higher quality of orientation as a means of improving their job satisfaction. Consecutive assignments was suggested by 33 percent of the dissatisfied nurses as compared to only 15 percent of the satisfied nurses. This finding coincides with the higher number of dissatisfied nurses desiring a limited number of areas for floating, indicating, perhaps, that stability in the work situation is important for their job satisfaction.

Although a high percentage of both groups of nurses listed having to reorient themselves to different areas as a disadvantage of floating, only 15 percent of the satisfied nurses and none of the dissatisfied nurses suggested standardization of units as to location of equipment and procedures. The investigator believes this incongruity was significant since the comments under Orientation specifically mentioned orienting

TABLE 3

Comparative Frequency and Percentage Distribution of Suggestions
for Improving Floating as Perceived by Satisfied
and Dissatisfied Nurses

Item	Frequency of Mention		Percentage Distribution	
	Satisfied Nurses	Dissatisfied Nurses	Satisfied Nurses, %	Dissatisfied Nurses, %
Limit number of areas to which a nurse will float	3	3	15	50
Higher quality of orientation	4	1	21	16
Consecutive assignment	3	2	15	33
Improve attitudes toward float nurse	2	1	10	16
Standardize location of equipment and procedures	3	-	15	-
Include float nurses in inservice	1	2	5	33
Evaluate utilization of float nurses	1	1	5	16

oneself to supplies and equipment and becoming familiar with routines, procedures, and idiosyncracies of the different units as a disadvantage. Only a few nurses indicated belief that eradication of that disadvantage would improve their job satisfaction.

The above findings correspond with those of Herzberg et al. and Friedlander in disproving the common assumption of a bipolar satisfaction-dissatisfaction continuum.[10,11] According to the bipolar continuum, respondents who find certain aspects of their jobs particularly important to their satisfaction would experience pronounced dissatisfaction when those elements were lacking in the job. The same could be said of the presence of dissatisfactory elements. That is, if certain elements of the job were particularly dissatisfying, the respondent would experience pronounced satisfaction if these elements were removed. Friedlander's study disproved the bipolar continuum of satisfaction and dissatisfaction, finding that respondents who believed certain aspects of the job particularly important to their satisfaction *did not* find the lack of or negative aspect of the same characteristics particularly important to their dissatisfaction. Similarly in this survey, although a majority of respondents listed orientation as a time-consuming disadvantage of floating, they did not suggest that measures to detensify this disadvantage would improve their job satisfaction.

Being included in workshops and inservice appeared to be more important to dissatisfied nurses (33 percent) than to satisfied nurses (0.5 percent); both groups, however, men-

tioned that improved attitudes of other staff toward the float nurse would add to their job satisfaction. Sixteen percent of the dissatisfied nurses and five percent of the satisfied nurses suggested that the utilization of the float nurse should be evaluated.

DISCUSSION

No attempt was made in this survey to determine why the respondents floated, if they preferred to float, or if they floated because they had no choice. One factor that could have influenced the responses was the unusually high number of nurses living in the geographic location for the survey. Because of the availability of nurses, there was a decreased possibility of being able to work straight shifts, especially days, except on a float basis, and floating provided one of the few work situations in which the nurse could set her own hours.

Smith proposed that job satisfaction is a function of the perceived characteristics of a job in relation to an individual's frame of reference.[12] In this respect job satisfaction could be related to the alternatives available to the individual. It is possible that, in view of the alternatives available to the float nurses in the survey, they could report satisfaction with floating in an effort to make the available position more desirable.

Vroom states that individual characteristics may condition reactions to different aspects of the work situation.[13] One such possibility is that individuals develop different adaptation levels or standards of judgment as a result of the differences in the amount or kind of experience in work situations. Thus, some may be easily satisfied, reporting satisfaction if the work situation meets certain minimal requirements, whereas others may have much higher thresholds for satisfaction. The significant response by satisfied nurses that "floating provides variety in the work situation and thus prevents boredom" could be an example of Vroom's proposition. Variety in the work situation could be the minimal requirement for job satisfaction. That is, if nurses find that floating satisfied a great need for variety, many of the disadvantages of floating could be overlooked. No attempt was made to determine the length of time each nurse had floated, or minimal requirements for their job satisfaction. It is possible, however, that float nurses do develop different levels of adaptation and standards of judgment regarding the float position.

The investigator noted that both the advantages and disadvantages listed were related to the frequent change of assignment inherent in the float position. That is, while floating produces a need for constant orientation—to different units, patients, staff, and physicians—creates insecurity in the float nurse, and deprives her of belonging to a specific work group, the respondents found the variety of work involved in floating to be stimulating.

The general findings of the survey support, in part, Bullock's study on the position, function, and job satisfaction of nurses.[14] He found that dissatisfactions appeared to be associated chiefly with social and organizational relationships. Of the disadvantages listed by both satisfied and dissatisfied nurses, six items were concerned with social and organizational relationships. These findings likewise lend support to the job satisfaction survey by Pickens and Tayback in which the staff nurse's relationship with her coworkers was found to be a vital force in job satisfaction.[15] The strong response by dissatisfied nurses regarding staff attitudes toward float nurses and being unfairly evaluated by peers indicates that these factors indeed may be a source of job dissatisfaction.

This survey did not fully support the findings of Smith's study dealing with job satisfaction of part-time nurses.[16] In that study the nurses were most satisfied with the quantity of supervision received, the manner in which their hours were scheduled, and the recognition they received. Job dissatisfaction was found to be related to matters of hospital policy and salary, lounge facilities, and fringe benefits. Since this investigator utilized open-ended questions in the survey, the subjects had complete freedom in their choice of response. The only item mentioned by the respondents that corresponded to Smith's study was that the flexible scheduling of hours was an advantage of floating. None of the other items contained in Smith's study were mentioned by either satisfied or dissatisfied float nurses.

CONCLUSIONS AND IMPLICATIONS

As indicated earlier, the pilot study was intended to provide information that could be utilized by directors of nursing service to promote job satisfaction for the professional float nurse. From the findings of the survey, several conclusions may have implications for nursing service. Although the majority of the float nurses included in the survey expressed satisfaction with floating, consideration should be given to the stated disadvantages of the float position and to the suggestions offered by these float nurses on how to improve their job satisfaction.

Even though both satisfied and dissatisfied nurses perceived the new learning and experience provided by floating as a distinct advantage, the need for constant orientation and reorientation seemed to be a source of strong dissatisfaction. Although a great deal of effort may already be directed to proper orientation of float nurses, this finding could indicate that present orientation practices may need to be reevaluated in terms of their effectiveness and relevancy for the float nurse.

Both satisfied and dissatisfied nurses expressed feelings of insecurity associated with floating, suggesting perhaps that further attention needs to be given to delineating those factors about floating which contribute most to the security and insecurity of the float nurse. Also, the challenge inherent in floating, of being able to adapt, did not appear to be a significant advantage for either group of nurses. In fact, both satisfied and dissatisfied nurses suggested limitation of the number of areas to which a nurse would float and consecutive assignments to the same area. It would seem that greater consideration might be given these factors in the assignment of float nurses and that such consideration might add to the security of the float nurse.

Although dissatisfied nurses seemed to experience a general lack of interest in becoming involved with others in the administrative aspects of the day-to-day functioning of the units, they did consider poor attitudes of staff toward float nurses as a distinct disadvantage of floating. The satisfied nurses also suggested that improvement of staff attitudes toward the float nurse would add to their job satisfaction. The strong response regarding poor attitudes of staff toward the float nurse could possibly indicate misguided staff expectations of the float nurse. Behavioral expression of poor attitudes and subsequent response to that behavior could carry over into the patient situation. Determination of staff expectations of the float nurse might possibly lead to a clarification of roles and responsibilities and a better understanding between the nurses involved.

The variety of work provided by floating was perceived as more of an advantage by satisfied nurses than by dissatisfied nurses, indicating the possibility that a need for variety and stimulation is a characteristic of nurses who enjoy floating. Recognition of individual preferences for variety or routine in assignments and in the selection of nurses for float duties might result in more satisfaction for those nurses who do float.

Finally, the findings of the preliminary survey suggest that further study may be useful in determining other factors regarding the float position that may influence the job satisfaction of the float nurse. Since greater numbers of health agencies are adopting the float position to provide for flexibility in staffing, it would seem that further study is warranted to ensure that flexibility is not obtained at the sacrifice of the personal job satisfaction for nurses assigned to the float position.

REFERENCES ON PAGE 52

REFERENCES

1. Brown, E.L. *Newer Dimensions of Patient Care, Part 2.* New York: Russell Sage Foundation, 1962, pp. 37-55.
2. Nahm, H. Job Satisfaction in Nursing. *American Journal of Nursing* 12:1389-1392, 1940.
3. Bullock, R. Position, Function and Job Satisfaction of Nurses in the Social System of a Modern Hospital. *Nursing Research* 2:4-14, 1953.
4. Pickens, M., and Tayback, M. A Job Satisfaction Survey. *Nursing Outlook* 5:157-159, 1957.
5. Maryo, J. and Lasky, J. A Work Satisfaction Survey Among Nurses. *American Journal of Nursing* 59:501, 1959.
6. Simon, R., and Olson, M. Assessing Job Attitudes of Nursing Service Personnel. *Nursing Outlook* 8:424-427, 1960.
7. Smith, M. A Study of the Extent of Job Satisfaction of a Group of Professional Nurses with Certain Factors Relative to Their Employment. Unpublished master's thesis, University of Colorado, 1963.
8. Selltiz, C., Jahoda, M., Deutsch, M., and Cook, S. *Research Methods in Social Relations, Part 2.* New York: The Dryden Press, 1951, pp. 423-462.
9. Brown, *loc. cit.*
10. Herzberg, M., and Snyderman, B. *The Motivation to Work.* New York: John Wiley & Sons, 1959.
11. Friedlander, F. Job Characteristics as Satisfiers and Dissatisfiers. *Journal of Applied Psychology* 48:388-392, 1964.
12. Smith, P., Kendall, L., and Hulin, C. *The Measurement of Satisfaction in Work and Retirement.* Chicago: Rand McNally, 1969, pp. 11-26.
13. Vroom, V. *Work and Motivation.* New York: John Wiley & Sons, 1964.
14. Bullock, *loc. cit.*
15. Pickens, Tayback, *loc. cit.*
16. Smith, M., *loc. cit.*

Maintaining the Job Performance of the Aging Employee

By Lawrence L. Steinmetz and R. Dennis Middlemist

Lawrence L. Steinmetz, Ph.D. is Professor of Management, University of Colorado Graduate School of Business Administration, Boulder, Colorado. **R. Dennis Middlemist,** Ph.D., is Assistant Professor of Organizational Behavior at the University of Wisconsin-Green Bay. The article is reprinted from JONA, March-April 9971.

As a person ages he undergoes a series of personality and attitudinal changes because he realizes his lifetime is nearing an end. The approach of retirement and the imminent loss of one's major role in life—the occupational role—influences a person's motivational pattern. He is less interested in advancement and in future goals.

The need for security and recognition increases as one grows older. The aging worker needs reinforcement, encouragement, and support. He is able to produce effectively, though at a slower pace, and properly motivated, he can contribute new ideas and be of benefit to the organization.

During the past several years there has been a marked increase in interest in the problems of aging and its impact on the performance of people at work. In part, this heightened concern over the problems of the aged is attributable to the increase in life expectancy, which has been responsible for a marked rise in the number of older people at work, and in part it has been in response to the observable phenomenon that as one ages, interests at work change.

The concept, "older worker," is a highly relative one. There are striking and significant differences from occupation to occupation, and from industry to industry, as to the age at which a person is considered to be an older worker. For instance, occupations which require great physical exertion, long hours or irregular hours, or are deemed hazardous, frequently limit employment to younger workers. Occupations which require long periods of training and experience are more likely to accept older workers. Obviously nursing and the whole profession of medical care falls in *both* categories.

It should therefore be beneficial to nursing administrators and supervisors to understand as much about the hospital work force as possible and how nurses' motivations to work change, in order to use fully the talents of the limited supply of trained hospital personnel available in the country. Studies by people such as Mayo and Herzberg have done much to show how to motivate employees, but there is reason to doubt that all these motivators are effective for older employees. For instance, since further promotion is usually only a remote possibility for the older employee, is self-actualization an effective motivator?

Should management encourage the older worker or simply make the best of a bad situation

This article will endeavor to answer the question of what can be done to motivate people as they grow older on the job, with special attention devoted to the problem as it applies to hospital employees. To answer this question, however, we must first answer the more basic question: How does a worker change in attitude and behavior as he ages? This question has vast implications for all managers, but especially for those in hospital and nursing home situations. If management can understand these changes, it can probably influence or cope with the changes brought on by employees' growing older. We will also try to answer some other questions: If the older worker is not susceptible to some motivators, might he be more susceptible to others? Is it worthwhile to try to encourage the older worker, or must management simply make the best of a bad situation because of social responsibility?

Changes in Personality and Attitude with Aging

Personality exercises a decisive influence on the way an individual accepts various motivations. It also is a crucial aspect of growing old. It is essential to examine changes in personality and self-concept of an aging individual if one is to comprehend fully the problem of the aging employee.

The personality of an individual is closely related to his attitudes and interests. What a person likes and dislikes, what he expresses as his attitude or feeling, is in essence his personality. An understanding of personality change might be obtained, then, by examining changes in attitudes and interests. This is also substantially easier than developing other types of personality studies.

Personality is, of course, developed while one is young and crystallizes as one grows old. For example, childhood is marked by a wide range of interests and much curiosity about the world. In adolescence these interests narrow and center upon a few specific activities.[1] What happens in maturity and old age?

One study, using the Strong vocational-interest questionnaire, shows that there is relatively little change in a person's main patterns of interest between the ages of twenty and sixty.[2] If he likes classical music at twenty, he will be likely to prefer it at sixty. If he likes numbers at twenty, math will interest him later on. However, a person also is not apt to develop any new interests after twenty. If a person doesn't like classical music at twenty, he probably won't care for it as he grows older either. The theory is basically that later vocational interests go back to patterns developed in adolescence.

There is a definite interpretation which may be made from this study, that there are distinct advantages in exposing the individual in childhood and youth to wide varieties of stimulation and experience in order that he may have the opportunity to locate areas of activity which can become permanent sources of interest. The wider the exposure, the more is the chance that the individual will develop those interests which bring him basic satisfaction.

It is desirable for people to determine their careers early in life—they are far more inclined to be content with their work. For example, from 1963 to 1965, Melzer[3] conducted research which indicated that attitude to work appears to be age-oriented. Generally, he found that satisfaction with one's work increased with age. The aging worker was less interested in promotion and more concerned about keeping a steady job. This might be true of the aging managerial employee also.

When older people look back on their past occupational experiences, achievement, recognition, and advancement stand out as the important satisfactions with their jobs. However, in their later years only the minor satisfactions of pay, interpersonal relations, supervision, and technical skills seem important to them. Both men and women exhibit this attitude toward work. Further, most older employees anticipate future problems with health and the need to keep busy, while the younger employees tend to expect problems in the job because of lack of recognition and achievement.

Another important change in the attitude of the aging worker is in the *quality* of interactions with subordinates. As an individual becomes middle-aged, he is more likely to change from concern with matters of welfare and human relations to a growing concern with the job itself. This may not be due to aging, per se, but to a change in responsibility, to past promotions, and present job position.[4]

Intelligence

Intelligence is another major factor in the motivation of people, but one which is usually not recognized by most supervisors. Difference in intelligence is one prime consideration in determining how far a person can go or what goals he should attempt to achieve. Intelligence also helps the person who is motivated to achieve his goals. Lack of intelligence or failing intelligence might hinder an individual's ambition. Intelligence is also crucial in developing ideas, which are the basis of regard and importance in an economic society.

K. W. Schaie[5] tested 500 people between the ages of twenty and seventy on factors of motor control, personality perception, and speed, to determine differences attributable to age. He found that spontaneous flexibility of ideas fell off *after the forties,* and that personality rigidity and the liking for a habit *increased continually from the twenties.* However, he feels there is some evidence to suggest that intelligence itself is the controlling factor, rather than increasing age.

What implications does this knowledge have for nursing administrators? It explains why some older people try to gravitate toward thinking jobs and why others staunchly avoid them. For example, it is known that people who age most successfully generally value wisdom more than physical powers. (Wisdom is distinguished from pure intellectual capacity as being the ability to make the most effective choice from a group of alternatives.) Many younger people begin their occupational careers in unskilled positions which require either great physical strength or, in a low-skilled job, great physical speed. But as one grows older, he inevitably experiences diminished physical ability and finds it increasingly difficult to meet the demands of a job. The critical transition point appears to be in the early forties.

Yet some people cling to these physical powers as their tools for coping with life because, as they see it, that is the way to stay young. These people, of course, have an attitude of repugnance toward aging. As a result, they become increasingly depressed, bitter, or otherwise unhappy as they age and are most likely to become problem employees. Conversely, those people who put the use of their heads above their hands are more interested in their work, are generally better adjusted, and usually pose fewer problems.

Intelligence, then, emerges as an important factor in determining whether the worker can continue to adapt to his environment as he grows older. It also helps determine another factor—his skill level, which is critical to any employee's performance at work. It can be stated as a general rule that the more intelligent older employee will be able to keep up with changing skill requirements. For example, psychologists are generally much more interested in the rate of learning than the capacity or quality of the learning. Employers, however, are much more concerned with the presence of the skill, e.g., whether the man or woman is an excellent surgical assistant, rather than how long it took him to learn the skills required. The importance of this difference can be spelled out as follows: persons above 45 years must spend from 15 to 20 percent more time in practice to acquire a new skill than persons at 18 or 19 years of age (which is about the age of maximum learning capacity).[6] But the difference is slight *in terms of actual performance* and is readily compensated for by a little extra effort and persistence upon the part of the older person. This factor becomes readily apparent when one thinks of older people who become interested in a hobby or task and devote great portions of time to learning what is required, and perform a remarkable job as a result.

His self-image may be undermined when he can no longer fulfill his occupational role

There are two factors which account for the older person's ability to keep up: motivation and practice. It is evident that there are two problems which the nursing administrator must be aware of in securing a good adjustment of the aging worker to the job environment. One is the problem of motivating him, helping him to see that he can learn, and building his interest in the new task. The other problem is to encourage him to give a little extra time and effort to build up to the level required in the new skill. The older worker will require more time to rid himself of the old habits and attitudes.

Role Perception—Its Impact Upon Performance

A perceived social role consists of the pattern of behavior expected of an individual taking part in a social or group situation. For example, the position of president of General Motors Corporation carries with it a set of duties, obligations, and rights, as does the position of resident or intern in a hospital. These duties, obligations, and rights constitute an expected behavior pattern for the person filling each position and he is expected to act according to the role he assumes.

Work is a major social role in our society. It may serve as the cornerstone of an individual's identity as well as proof of his competence and worth. Thus, any man or woman's self-image may be seriously undermined when he or she is no longer able, or allowed, to fulfill his occupational role.

As a worker becomes older, he is often prevented, either by health or by administrative fiat, from full participation in his occupational role. The loss of the identity of his occupational role can have serious influence upon the worker's motivation. He might exhibit one of three reactions: he may withdraw or become introspective and no longer identify himself with the job, thereby establishing a new role for himself; he may look forward to retirement and, in fact, identify with that role and no longer feel the need to excel in his job; or he may become more motivated, pushing himself beyond his normal capacity to work in an attempt to preserve his occupational role.

Reactions to Aging

An important theory has been advanced in recent years to explain or describe the process by which people adjust to the fact of aging. Elaine Cumming and William Henry have called theirs the "theory of disengagement."[7] Essentially, the theory is that, as a person ages, he begins to accept the inevitability of death and begins preparing for it by gradual withdrawal from some of his societal roles. Disengagement is the process in which many of the relationships of the individual and society are severed, and other social roles are altered.

In our society, success is judged on the basis of skill and knowledge (the occupational role). But, according to social beliefs, age is usually accompanied by declining knowledge and skill, so there are societal pressures on the aging worker to disengage himself from his occupational role. By the same token, as the individual ages, his self-concept is altered. He is likely to perceive his knowledge and skill as declining and may begin the disengagement process himself.

The way in which a person adapts to the aging process depends largely on his personality—on dominant needs, defenses, and adaptive mechanisms. How well he adjusts to growing older depends on whether or not he can meet his needs and defend his current situation. Good social adjustment for the older worker is primarily a matter of how well he has been able to assimilate his past experiences and be satisfied by his total value or contributions.

There are important differences in the goals of older persons, however. The ages at which individuals give up their dominant roles will vary greatly from one person to another. It would seem reasonable to expect that people who, when younger, were active in planning, were long-range-goal oriented and were rewarded for this, would continue this orientation much further into old age than would other individuals. Eventually, the aging process and other external factors will reduce the realistic possibilities for planning for future goals, and even optimistic individuals will gradually disengage.

An important factor in the aging process is the changing time perspective that occurs as age increases. The awareness of age by an individual increases his awareness of time past and diminishes his willingness to look ahead. In early childhood, the psychological future is vague and poorly structured; in adolescence the future is seen as limitless. At about the age of thirty the individual recognizes that time and life are finite. This, then, becomes the age of great motivation, when the individual is concerned with expansion. Goals become specific and activities toward these goals become more significant. In later years the recognition comes that the time available for life is now seriously limited. Setbacks are more serious and, when they occur, cause an increasing need to conserve and protect against loss. This is why many workers develop negative motivations, increasing their need for security and increasing their susceptibility to threats or imagined threats. To protect his job, a worker may feel his old skill is what he is needed for, and *he may be hesitant to learn new skills* at which he may not be as efficient and hence, not as needed. Or he may take care not to over produce, thereby insuring that no layoff will come from over production.

Retirement

The period when a worker nears the age of retirement is a critical period of social adaption. Physical decline, made apparent by approaching retirement age, portends the approach of death. This prospect may even take on unreal proportions for those working in medicine, especially among the aged in nursing homes. Further, a series of rapid changes in expected social behavior undermine a worker's sense of identity at this age. Because one's occupational role is one of the most important social roles in defining identity, retirement, with its implications of uselessness, is a focal event which typifies the problems of aging.

Faced with retirement and in an unstable social position, an individual may respond in various ways. The two prevalent attitudes which a worker may adopt are: to accept the inevitability of retirement and its implications of old age, or to ignore the approaching disaster and try to work beyond the age of retirement.

Research in the field of psychology indicates that those workers who welcome retirement and can adjust to the fact of aging or approaching death, are those who generally are satisfied with their life's accomplishments in the occupational role. If a worker feels he has achieved realistic accomplishments in terms of his abilities and goals, he is likely to be satisfied with other goals and will look forward to retirement.

However, many workers are not satisfied with their accomplishments and feel frustrated with their loss of identity. Generally, these workers feel it is important to keep their hands busy, frequently commenting that idleness leads to physical or mental deterioration and death. Though they may not be motivated to accomplish more at work, they are nevertheless reluctant to give up the occupational role because they must then face the nearness of death.

Motivation

In analyzing the effects of aging on the motivation to work of hospital and nursing personnel, we must take into account several different but related changes in individual psychological development. Throughout the process of maturity and old age, many changes take place which alter a person's values and attitudes. As one grows older, he wants different things from life. Concerns about physical appearance, standard of living, and family matters change. Motivation (drive), in general, tends to decrease. Older workers have less intense enthusiasm and frequently need strong incentives, support, and encouragement to accomplish tasks which would have thrilled them in years past. Older workers are greatly concerned about preserving the gains they have made in their lifetimes and hence are not disposed to take new risks which might threaten their past rewards.

Older workers are an important asset . . . they have much to contribute

The younger worker is strongly motivated by a desire to accomplish those life goals which he has set out for himself. He is additionally motivated by his responsibility to his wife and children and the regard of his neighbors, and is spurred by competition with his fellow workers. He receives cross stimulation from other persons—clergymen, parents, interested friends, etc.—which reinforces his primary motivations.

For the older person these motivations are seriously weakened. He has generally accomplished the goals which he had established earlier, his family responsibilities are much less, and he is no longer concerned with impressing his neighbors. The motivation of the older worker is determined by his immediate needs and desires, his tendency towards loneliness, his feeling of uselessness, and his need for support.

Three factors which are important in understanding how an individual reacts to incentives (or how he can be motivated) are: the individual's perception of the nature of the external environment, his inner motivation, and his action initiation. A study, cited by John E. Anderson in the book,

Psychological Aspects of Aging, reveals the differences in these three factors in relation to age.[8]

The individual's perception of the nature of the external environment, the world around him, varies greatly with age. In his thirties a person has an easy and confident attitude toward the outside world. He feels it can be dealt with; no problem is insurmountable. In the decade of his forties, the outer world begins to take on life and complexity for the individual, and he begins to be aware of his inner motivations. After fifty he has a greater interest in a wider social orbit. He is more aware of a potentially malign outer world, one that can take away as well as give.

The younger person, in his thirties, feels his inner life is essentially a threat to his ambitions and goals, hence he denies his inner desires. At forty his inner motivation becomes a source of concern and conflict, and by fifty he may become quite introspective. He is apt to examine his self concept and develop those non-monetary goals he previously denied.

Action initiation is the extent to which a person perceives himself as able to direct and influence actions and things around him. In his thirties, a person is likely to be bound by stereotypes and the necessity of following directions issued by others. By his forties one's action initiation is most pronounced; he is more confident of his directing and influencing abilities. As a result of his past experiences, the individual in his fifties is overwhelmed by the wide range of possibilities and alternatives in the world. He has less interest in influencing these possibilities, will settle for less, and set no new goals for himself.

These differences in the three factors correspond to the studies previously mentioned in aging, roles, and retirement. Although a number of studies show a general increase in job satisfaction with an increase in age, there is evidence to the contrary.

In 1955, a study by Turner showed workers may begin to feel hopeless as they contemplate growing older in a job which holds little interest for them.[9] This study showed the level of satisfaction among managers increased continually from about twenty-nine to fifty-nine, but declined at sixty (pre-retirement years). The decline was probably also caused by actual or anticipated blocking of channels for self-actualization; because of the managers' age, companies do not give them opportunities for further advancement or achievement. It is quite conceivable that the decline in satisfaction is due to changes in the individual's inner motivation or action initiation.

The problem of motivation in the elderly is also complicated by social demands, feedback, and reinforcements. These change motivational problems. The elderly are worried about making fools of themselves in the presence of their group and may act abnormally in very ordinary situations. Nonetheless, it can be generally stated that motivational changes due to aging are: the avoidance of risk, less action toward meeting challenges, and the tendency towards introspection.

Individual Differences

There is always a danger in speaking about general reactions as if all persons were alike. People are not identical and often not even similar. Therefore, we must be careful to be aware of the existence of individual differences.

Despite the vast implications of growing old, it is clear that individuals react quite differently to the whole process of growing older. The variations cannot be explained in terms of different social status. While there is evidence of differences in the reactions of different social groups (i.e., doctors compared to custodians), there is also evidence of differences in individuals within social groups. Two older workers doing identical tasks may view the task quite differently. One may still feel challenged by the job, while the other may be bored or frustrated. For example, one nurse may be a problem and another of the same age no problem whatsoever.

It is reasonable to assume that these differences may be because of deep-seated personality differences or differences in self-concept. While there is some truth that older workers, as a group, tend to be more set in their ways, many older persons *are* adaptable, and have demonstrated this successfully by making significant contributions to society, late in life.

Implications

What slows down the aging employee? It is clear that it is not deteriorating health, in most instances, but rather a number of psychological factors. The older worker wants to work, even though he may be satisfied with his past accomplishments. Work is important to him as a foundation of self-respect and a source of prestige. It provides an opportunity for social interaction and discourages self preoccupation.

The worker may become bored with his achievements; if he has a relatively secure income, the job will begin to lose its challenge for him.

In addition to the lack of challenge, the successful older person lacks recognition and is taken for granted. There is also a feeling that men and women at fifty-five are over the hill. Administrators often forget that the experience of these older employers can be extremely valuable to younger personnel. What better way to motivate successful older people than by having them serve as mentors wherever possible, offering them a new challenge of value to the organization. Consider them experts to be consulted when difficult problems arise. Show them you recognize their past contributions and still expect new ones. Use their abilities and experiences in the assistance of others. Such new tasks will not destroy their feelings of security, which would be based on the same foundation of past experiences that they used in performing the old duties. The new possibilities for self-esteem and sense of worth in attempting new duties will be effective motivators.

Summary

In modern industry, business, and society as a whole, individuals have tended to be cut off from work opportunities as they approach the age of retirement. The trend has been the same in hospitals and nursing homes. The reasoning is that the older worker is not as productive, not as physically fit, and does not react readily to incentives. The older worker is accused of being set in his ways and often of being senile. It is perhaps too easy to generalize about the old worker.

Actually, only 2 percent of people over sixty-five are bedridden, and relatively few are senile.[10] The problem of motivation in the older worker is not one of senility, but has to do with the whole range of effects that the aging process has on an individual.

When a person is younger, he experiences the normal motivations of accomplishment, family responsibility, and the need for esteem. The normal individual seeks in some way to show his superiority over other human beings. He craves recognition, distinction, success, power, leadership, wealth, and influence. He considers himself to be the best of the group.

However, as the individual ages he undergoes profound personality changes. Although he is not likely to develop new interests he may cultivate some old ones which he has never had the opportunity to do so before. Interests and attitudes become determined, but the individual can still learn.

Even though the rate of learning decreases with age (after eighteen) the capacity to learn is still strong in the older worker. Properly motivated, the older employee can learn new tasks, new methods and be a productive worker. The older employee is likely to adopt a belief in the use of his brain, rather than his brawn, to cope with problems.

The primary blockade to successful motivation is threatened security, because the aging worker fears his loss of identity as he sees his occupational role lessen. He is expected to disengage from the role which has been most important to him throughout his life. The adjustments which the individual must make are great. Some individuals adapt quite well, while others do not. The differences are attributable to differences in personality characteristics, attitudes and interests.

It is difficult to generalize about motivational changes caused by the aging process. Motivation in general (drive) tends to decrease. Some kinds of motivational changes may be true for some persons, but not for others. Age changes in motivation are very much a matter of development, depending on past experiences in life, and the individual's reaction as he realizes life's end is near.

Evidence has shown that the older worker is still susceptible to such motivators as the need for security and recognition, although some individuals no longer need further advancement. It has been found that older workers are an important asset to administrators because of their long experience. Since older workers constitute a sizeable proportion of the work force, and since older workers still have much to contribute, it behooves nursing administrators to attempt to motivate those individuals who have adapted well to the aging process.

BIBLIOGRAPHY

ANDERSON, JOHN E. *Psychological Aspects of Aging.* Washington, D.C., American Psychological Association, Division on Maturity and Old Age, 1956.

ANDERSON, JOHN E. *The Psychology of Development and Personal Adjustment.* New York, Henry Holt & Co., 1949.

BROMLEY, D. B. *The Psychology of Human Aging.* Baltimore, Penguin Books, Inc., 1966.

GEIST, HAROLD. *The Psychological Aspects of Retirement.* Springfield, Ill., Charles C. Thomas, Pub., 1968.

LOETHER, HERMAN J. *Problems of Aging.* Belmont, Cal., Dickenson Pub. Co., Inc., 1967.

REICHARD, SUZANNE. *Aging and Personality.* New York, John Wiley & Sons, Inc., 1962.

SALCH, SHOUKEY D. "Age and Level of Job Satisfaction." *Personnel Psychology,* 17, Winter 1964.

SCHAIE, K. WARNER. *Theory and Methods of Research on Aging.* Morgantown, W. Va., West Virginia University, 1968.

TRYTTEN, J. M. "How to Motivate the Older Salesman." *Inland Printer/American Lithographer,* 161, May 1968.

WILLIAMS, C. "What About the Older Workers." *Supervisory Management,* 12, Sept. 1967.

REFERENCES

1. ANDERSON, JOHN E. *The Psychology of Development and Personal Adjustment.* New York, Henry Holt & Co., 1949, p. 534.
2. ANDERSON, *Development,* p. 535.
3. SCHAIE, K. WARNER. *Theory and Methods of Research on Aging.* Morgantown, W. Va., West Virginia University, 1968, p. 154.
4. SCHAIE, *Research on Aging,* p. 139.
5. *Ibid.* p. 152.
6. ANDERSON, *Development,* p. 526.
7. LOETHER, HERMAN J. *Problems of Aging.* Belmont, Cal., Dickenson Pub. Co., Inc., 1967, p. 19.
8. ANDERSON, JOHN E. *Psychological Aspects of Aging.* Washington, D.C., American Psychological Association, Division on Maturity and Old Age, 1956.
9. REICHARD, SUZANNE. *Aging and Personality.* New York, John Wiley & Sons, Inc., 1962, p.2.
10. REICHARD, *Aging,* p. 5.

Library of Congress Catalog Card Number: 74-76942
International Standard Book Number: 0-913654-01-9

Bibliography

Beltzhoover, M., (1994). Self-Scheduling: An Innovative Approach. <u>Nursing Management</u>, 25(4), 81-82.

Brusco, M.J., Futch, J., & Showalter, M.J. (1993). Staff Planning Under Conditions of a Nursing Shortage. <u>Journal of Nursing Administration</u>, 23(7/8), 58-64.

Curtin, L., (1993). Keepers of the Keys: Economics, ethics, and nursing administrators. <u>Nursing Administration Quarterly</u>, 17(4), 1-10.

Segesten, K., Agelii, E., Elmcrona, M., Lindstrom, I., & Lundren, S. (1994). Nurses' experience of change: A new professional collaboration model and all RN staffing. <u>Nursing Administraion Quarterly</u>, 18(4), 72-78.

Staff(1993, January). Fighting Staff Cuts, California RNs Push for Enforceable Patient Ratios. <u>American Journal of Nursing</u>, p81.

Wieseke, A., & Bantz, D. (1992). Economic Awareness of Registered Nurses Employed in Hospitals. <u>Nursing Economics</u>, 10(6), 406-412.